D1253257

Traumatic Brain Injury: TBI

&

Post-Concussion Syndrome: PCS

10 Simple Steps
Your Doctor May Not Know
That Can Help You

C. Rae Johnson

Copyright © 2017 by C. Rae Johnson
All rights reserved. No part of this publication may be reproduced, stored in a retrieval system, or transmitted in any form by any means, electronic, mechanical, photocopy, recording, or otherwise, without the prior written permission of author.

All rights reserved. Use by permission.
craejohnsonfaithbasedbooks@gmail.com

Cover design: John Johnson
  Image: Copyright: <a href='https://www.123rf.com/profile_woodoo007'>woodoo007 / 123RF Stock Photo</a>

First printing 2017
Printed in the United States of America

Scripture quotations are taken from the King James Version of the Holy Bible, New Living Translation and the New American Standard Bible.

"Scripture quotations taken from the New American
Standard Bible® (NASB),
Copyright © 1960, 1962, 1963, 1968, 1971, 1972,
1973, 1975, 1977, 1995 by The Lockman Foundation
Used by permission. www.Lockman.org"

Scripture quotations are taken from the Holy Bible, New Living Translation, copyright ©1996, 2004, 2007, 2013, 2015 by Tyndale House Foundation. Used by permission of Tyndale House Publishers, Inc., Carol Stream, Illinois 60188. All rights reserved.

Information within this book is for educational purposes only. It is not intended to replace your physician or medical care. Please see your health-care provider before beginning suggestions in this book or any new health program; for complete well-being.

ISBN 978-1-365-79535-0

<ins>*All Scripture is Given for Instruction*</ins>

Scripture quotations marked KJV are taken from the King James Version Bible

Scripture quotations marked NASB are taken from the New American Standard Bible

Scripture quotations marked NLT are taken from the New Living Translation Bible

In honor of my Heavenly Father in Jesus Name

Dedication

This book is dedicated to my Heavenly Father through our Lord and Savior Jesus Christ and to all brain injured individuals and their families; as we are all striving to live our lives in this world together, struggling through the healing process. May we hold within ourselves and display to others the kind of comfort, hope, kindness and love we all so desperately need.

A very special loving and heartfelt thanks to my supportive and encouraging husband John and my wonderful children for allowing me the time to accomplish this feat of writing, in spite of my injury; all for the hopes of helping someone else. This surely has been an awe-inspiring and amazing journey and I truly appreciate the time and support as well as all of the love, comfort and guidance throughout the entire process. I love you all!

An extra special thank you to my darling husband John, for his creative expertise in his cover design and picture placement. It is beautifully worth the struggle. Thanks babe! I love you with an ongoing and endearing love.

Table of Contents

Introduction 13

1-Physical Needs 21

2-Nutrition & Supplements 41

3-Therapies 49

4-Sound & Noise Intolerance 57

5-Sight & Light Intolerance 61

6-Memory Lapses 69

7-Exercise 77

8-Moods & Emotions 105

9-Support Groups 117

10-Prayer & Meditation 125

Afterward 135

Notes 139

Acknowledgments

A special appreciative and heartfelt thank you for my dear friend Katy Whitton, for helping me to pull it all together through her editing expertise. Her continued help and support is just priceless and absolutely shows how God weaves people and circumstances together for a reason. I am very grateful for her in my life as she is highly respected and loved as a dear sister in Christ.

I am thankful for my injury and for the many doctors throughout, especially those who were helpful and also those of whom were not; as they only served to propel me to keep searching for the right answers, the right doctors and the most helpful therapies and in the process, I was able to increase my faith in a higher power.

I would like to extend an enduring thanks to my friend Eric Fiorillo at Fiorillo Barbell Company for suggesting one-sided training to me in the hopes of helping increase brain function and repair. I always enjoy our sharing exchange of helpful information and stories that increase our inspiration for endurance of both brain and brawn on the informative podcasts hosted by Eric Fiorillo.

http://motivationandmuscle.com/
https://fiorillobarbellco.com/

I would like to present a personal thank you to Dr. Raymond Delucci of Delucci Chiropractic for offering the help I needed both in relieving certain headache pain and spinal misalignment due to the brain injury and also for his supportive help in finding me a very helpful and conscientious family doctor; which set the stage to finally move forward with the right specialty doctors, testing, diagnostic blood work and treatments needed. It all starts with one caring person just willing to help and Dr. Delucci along with his wife Madeline and his family run practice is wonderful in their caring approach for the treatment of others.

website: http://deluccichiro.com email:

Drdelucci@DelucciChiro.com

https://www.facebook.com/Delucci-Chiropractic190466280974755/

I would also like to extend a very warm thank you to a dear friend and brother in Christ, Steve Olejar, who so graciously shared alternative therapies that were of help for him in coping with his battle with Traumatic Brain Injury and Post-Concussion Syndrome. Sharing helpful insights with one another is a great way to continue to increase hope; along with knowing that God ultimately has this, as well as us all.

Traumatic Brain Injury: TBI

&

Post-Concussion Syndrome: PCS

10 Simple Steps

Your Doctor May Not Know

That Can Help You

Introduction

There are absolutely some life events that we are not only never prepared for, but also do not fully understand; one of them being head injuries. Although oftentimes misdiagnosed and misunderstood a Traumatic Brain Injury, otherwise known as a TBI, is a head injury or concussion that is caused by a blow, bump, or jolt to the head that disrupts the normal functioning of the brain. Injuries range from a mild to a more severe form of brain injury acting as a neurological disease or disorder, with many symptoms affecting the injured person as a whole.

TBI is not only caused by an open head injury as in the case of a penetrating head wound, but also can be the result of a closed head injury as in a bump or a quick moving jolt. TBI's are the leading cause of death and disability, including the leading cause of seizures, contributing to approximately thirty percent of all injury deaths of the almost two million new cases reported each year. Those surviving TBI's can suffer effects ranging from as little as a few days, upwards to a lifetime of disabilities; leading to a syndrome known as Post-Concussion Syndrome or PCS.

PCS is an ongoing chronic syndrome of experiencing persistent, lingering concussion-like symptoms from a TBI or concussion injury that may develop due to the many risk factors involved, such as older age and gender (as females over 40 years of age are especially at a higher risk), multiple head injuries, and lack of rest. Up to 80% of concussions or Traumatic Brain Injuries will result in Post-

Concussion Syndrome. It is essential to obtain prompt treatment, adequate rest, proper nutrition, and the utilization of therapeutic therapies to help minimize the debilitating effects and possibly shorten the duration of the symptomatic experiences.

The debilitating effects encompass many bodily systems as connections, (the synapses between the neurons), are lost due to stretched or severed axons within the brain. Locating the site of impact and which lobes were damaged, can help determine symptoms and the length of the recovery process.

Don't forget that the brain is the body's computer system for all bodily functions, so depending on the point of impact and the severity of localized damage, we can begin to both understand and help gauge the recovery process through treatment specific therapy. Impairment can include physical, cognitive, behavioral/emotional, sensory and even result in personality changes which can either be subtle as in a hidden injury, or quite severely noticeable at times. As education grows about the tremendous impact a head or brain injury can have, not only on the person injured, but also for the caregivers, doctors, and families as well, we can all become more knowledgeable.

Some specific symptoms for Cognitive impairment include: slowed response time, mental fogginess, poor concentration, easily distracted, trouble with memory and learning, disorganization, difficulty problem solving and recognizing simple tasks; all of which can be extremely debilitating and frustrating.

Physical symptoms can include: headache, nausea, visual disturbances, light sensitivity, double vision, noise sensitivity, tinnitus, heightened sense of smell and sound, vertigo, balance disruptions, proprioception difficulties, hyper-vigilance, touch sensitive, dream-state feeling, lack of energy, fatigue, exhaustion, hormonal imbalances and sleep disturbances.

Behavioral changes can include: panic attacks, anxiety, depression, irritability, increased emotional responses such as anger or sudden crying, apathy, personality changes, and lowered tolerances to frustrations (easily frustrated).

These symptoms are many yet are not all of what can be experienced by a brain injured individual. It is estimated that 5.3 million Americans are living with disabilities related to brain injuries; although I personally believe that number to be in reality, much higher. I notice new people every day wanting to join brain injury support groups.

Recovering from a brain injury can be so much more complex depending on the severity of the impact than anyone can ever realize, unless you're actually experiencing it. If anyone you know of is going through such a life altering trauma, even if it's yourself, be extra, extra patient. It takes a long time for complete healing; and sometimes that may not even be possible. Some days you may feel absolutely great with next to no symptoms, because they seem so minor that it may feel like you're almost normal again and can tackle almost anything; that is until you start to venture out to do just that. Then you are reminded of your limits in a very profound way and may wonder if you will ever regain completeness or wholeness again.

What you do not know about yourself, you will begin to learn as this is just the start. For now, you do need to focus on just accepting where you are at, at this particular point in time; especially for the sake of your own sanity. Your brain needs any energy you have to heal, so fighting against where you are at in life right now will not help you in any way, but only hinder the healing process. Rather let go, accept and learn to love the new you. Accept any help and love from others as well, throughout your journey.

During your healing process you may become so overwhelmed, that you won't know what to do next, especially if you cannot do what you did before. You may find that you can't always rely on others to understand, when you yourself do not fully understand. So before the paralysis of defeat sets in, with the overwhelming stimuli always at your door, understand that just taking one step at a time can greatly lessen any feeling of anxiety or fear. Also learn to recognize those emotions for what they are; very unreliable. Know that they can just add to the confusion. If you can learn to seek light in your darkness and to cast out any fear or anxiety that tries to creep in, you're on your way to acceptance, because light casts out dark, and that involves fear, which includes fear of the unknown; such as what the future may now hold. Learn to just focus on the day at hand and only the next thing; that one thing that you can do, as you let the others just drift away for now. You will find hope as you see a light through the tunnel of this all-encompassing injury.

It is helpful to view this whole life circumstance from a different perspective with the replacement of thought processes, by removing all of the "I can't do's" in your life now...to the "I can do's" and the "I get to's". You may not be able to put yourself in situations that will ultimately result in too much stimuli, for instance, even driving may be extremely challenging and therefore dangerous if it brings on symptoms; which will be hard especially if you like your independence and the ability to just go.

But once your acute symptoms are managed, you do get to relax more, catch up on small house projects (it doesn't matter if you forget how...the point is the effort you are trying to make), meditate (on God's word if you're a believer, as it will definitely serve to strengthen you), sleep more, spend more quality down time at home with family; i.e. your spouse, kids and pets, et cetera. You will finally have the time to try a new creative project at your own pace. You can exercise slowly to increase your strength, flexibility and endurance once again, while both knowing your respectable limits, being ever watchful and mindful of your threshold; plus, it can help make those needed brain connections. Additionally, you may finally have the time to do something that you have always wanted to do for instance, writing, drawing/sketching, painting, gardening, et cetera, but were always too busy or too preoccupied to tackle. Just don't feel like you're missing out on a lot of things because maybe someday you will be busy again wishing you had this extra time back. Having the time to newly refresh yourself in life, even if it's challenging and frustrating at first, will show great growth as you learn and relearn your life with a whole new appreciation.

You can use this trial in your life to relate to others and any limitations that they might have, whether physically or mentally; especially concerning movements with daily activities, exercise, memory difficulties, or pain as in the form of headaches and migraines. Nutrition is such a huge part of the healing process as your body needs proper nutrition for the repair and healing process to begin; needing the nutrients that act as neuro-protectors for damaged neurons. It takes about two years for the brain to heal. With that being said, sometimes some people may have symptoms that last much longer and become ongoing. Every brain injury is different and cannot be explained as a textbook case, as there are just too many factors and variables involved including one's environment and lifestyle both before and after injury. As diverse and unique as any person is, so are their brain injuries.

I myself happen to fall into the category of a lengthy trial with ongoing symptoms, but rather than giving in or succumbing to defeat, wallowing in my misery as in mourning the "old" me, I choose to embrace the "new" me, by getting to know me now, with all of the new exciting and enjoyable things that I get to do. It is about learning to get passed the "self" in yourself, to stop looking inward to find the good out of it all.

It is about being thankful where you are at and being hopeful for your bright future. It's about learning that there is something more, a much bigger picture. Now I am a woman of faith so personally I never cease in prayer because I need something more; I need God and His strength to just get me through this daily. I believe, with knowledge in my heart that my Lord understands, He comforts me, gives me the grace and strength that I so desperately need to continue to just move forward, to just keep going because I've been at the bottom where there was nowhere but up. My personal testimony just shows that He will never leave you nor forsake you. That's a promise! So never give up! You're not alone in this. Your future is not yet fully written, for your "Story" may be just beginning. Just remember that you can press forward past this. You can keep going. Ultimately, you can persevere!

Don't be afraid, for I am with you. Don't be discouraged, for I am your God. I will strengthen you and help you. I will hold you up with my victorious right hand. Isaiah 41:10 NLT

And He said, "My presence shall go with you, and I will give you rest." Exodus 33:14 NASB

1

<u>Physical Needs</u>

Rest & Sleep: After such a traumatic injury as a brain injury, your body needs adequate rest to heal properly. Initially after the emergency room treatment, for the first few days, just rest. If you have a family member or friend to help, have them try to arouse or awake you from sleeping several times; every 3-4 hours for the first 24-48 hours, to reduce the complications that may occur. If there are any developing signs of deterioration in your mental status, go immediately to the hospital for further treatment as every moment counts for brain injury recovery.

Signs include:

Headache that worsens

Extremely drowsy and cannot be aroused or awakened

Difficulty recognizing people

Vomiting

Confusion and very irritable

Seizures

Bleeding from ears

Weakness and numbness

Unsteady and unbalanced gait (balance off)

Slurred speech

Or just not behaving and reacting as normal self.

Remember this is a hidden injury and not all symptoms may be displayed for others to see, as they can be very subtle.

After the initial 2-3 days pass you may start to notice having continual sleep disturbances; either of difficulty falling asleep or waking often while trying to maintain sleep. Take note of how often this occurs; talk with your doctor.

Sleep Disturbance: Oftentimes there is an associated sleep disturbance where there may be difficulty in sleeping related to head injuries. Melatonin is a hormone that helps to adjust the body's internal clock by regulating the sleep cycles, therefore it is used to aide in sleep disturbances. Melatonin has also been found useful in helping minimize brain swelling when given early on in a Traumatic Brain Injury. It is available both by prescription or over the counter. As always, check with your doctor first before taking this or any medicine or supplement as they may not be safe for everybody. There are some side-effects and should not be taken during pregnancy.

Not having adequate rest time after a Traumatic Brain Injury to enable your body to heal properly can increase your chances for developing Post-Concussion Syndrome.

PCS is an ongoing syndrome of experiencing persistent lingering concussion-like symptoms from a TBI that may develop due to risk factors involved such as age, gender (females over 40 years of age especially have a higher risk), multiple head injuries, and lack of rest.

Both physical rest combined with cognitive rest are important. Too much stimuli, even for concentration and focused attention, may exacerbate symptoms as well as be extremely draining, causing fatigue. Gradually return to activities of exercise or play when symptoms are cleared. If symptoms return upon activity this means it is time to rest again. Listen to your body's needs. If your body requires more rest, then take the time to do just that to avoid a relapse in your healing process. Stimuli can compound making some days worse than others. Daily exertion or stimuli experienced in one day may require more rest the next day. It just takes time; a lot of time so relax in the down time that you are given. Important...rest is preparation for renewal. Remember back when you may have wished for more time to just relax, well here you have it, so just make the most of it in the best way possible. You will grow in ways other than just making new connections in the brain, surprisingly in many others as well.

Headaches: Headaches and various degrees of head pain are more than common, they just seem to attack the brain at any given moment, as do the variable migraines that just seem to come out of nowhere; but is always unwelcomed with a "No, not now!" response. Plus, you may find that higher heat temperatures play a significant role in headaches causing an increase in frequency and sometimes even more pronounced in intensity. Headaches can vary in pain sensations from burning, sharpness, pressure, crushing and even may feel as though your head is open and present a "wet" sensation. Talking to your doctor about the exact sensations you are experiencing can help rule out complications. He may send you for an MRI (Magnetic Resonance Imaging) or more detailed scans as they can reveal vascular damage of lesions and any hemorrhaging within the brain. Keeping a headache journal will help you keep track of the types and location of head pain as it may fluctuate daily.

If you need to take a pain medication for headaches, choose a nonsteroidal anti-inflammatory medication such as ibuprofen (Motrin or Advil) rather than acetaminophen (Tylenol) due to the neurotoxicity it caused in mice and further inducing brain damage as announced in laboratory testing by the National Institutes of Health. Ibuprofen has also been shown to minimize TBI symptoms in other studies. Fortunately, NSAID's such as ibuprofen can help most head pain in moderation but be sure to eat when taking this medication as they can be more of an irritant to your stomach lining to the point of being dangerous by causing bleeding ulcers if taken without food for extended periods of time.

If you prefer to choose natural ways to relieve head pain, which is always better anyway, another helpful aide especially useful in helping migraine sufferers is a nutritional supplement, with its complete core nutrition being from a plant called moringa-oleifera. This is my personal preference of choice as it is medicinal grade quality, the freshest and oxidation-free. Moringa is considered to be the most nutrient dense plant that offers many health benefits with its naturally occurring anti-oxidants, anti-inflammatories, omegas, all essential amino acids, vitamin and mineral content, and is available through Green Virgin Products. Here is a quick link @ http://www.greenvirginproducts.com?aff=112

Moringa does the trick of knocking my migraines right out, stops them in their tracks (both the headache and the light disturbances).

Moringa is mentioned in the nutrition section as well because it is just so nutrient dense and beneficial to the human body for health and well-being. Our diets are usually lacking in nutrition as they are highly processed and inflammatory. So, although we eat for nutrition as well as hunger purposes, if we do not get enough nutritional value in our foods, our bodies will still be starving, even though we may be full. This is why we often keep searching for something else to eat, to gain that nutrition we are missing in our diets.

Certain types of headaches can also be relieved by chiropractic care as there could be muscle and soft tissue damage as well as misalignment of the spine due to the head injury. Seeking a chiropractor that can help alleviate the pressure on the nerves caused by the damage from injury, can offer some relief with headache pain.

Balance & Dizziness: Laying down for a rest really helps in the acute phases of dizziness and vertigo. For more chronic dizziness, first have a physician rule out any cervical spine or neck injuries. You can also have a physical therapist or inner ear doctor that specializes in Traumatic Brain Injury, monitor your dizziness by checking for calcium crystals in your inner ear canal that sometimes form due to head injuries. Having calcium crystals can cause a great deal of vertigo with feelings of the room spinning, that can appear suddenly with quick movements, such as sitting up from a lying down position too quickly. If inner ear crystals are suspected from a TBI you may be referred to an otologist or a neurotologist for an evaluation as they specialize in ear and brain connections. Here is a YouTube link for a quick exercise that may help eliminate or at least lesson the vertigo by moving the crystals in the canal that cause the disruption, by Dr. Carol Foster MD. https://www.youtube.com/watch?v=mQR6b7CAiqk&feature=youtu.be

Treatment for balance and vertigo is available through physical therapy by means of Vestibular Rehabilitation Therapy, which helps by improving equilibrium and balance that may be contributing to dizziness. It works by using specific eye, head and body exercises that are designed to retrain the brain to help it to recognize and process information or signals from the vestibular system, then coordinate the information from your vision and proprioception.

Proprioception: Proprioception is the sense and awareness of our body parts in relation to the world around us, orienting us to time and space of our surroundings, in so doing relates to balance in how we perceive our environment. It is essentially our body knowing where it is at in our environment. We have proprioceptors within our muscles, ligaments, tendons, and other soft tissues that act as tiny sensors which relay information to the brain regarding position, pressure and muscle stretching. They are specialized sensory receptors on nerve endings within these structures that send information to the brain, which the brain then reacts by positioning the body accordingly.

Sometimes with brain injuries, the proprioception will be off due to damage to these nerve endings resulting in an impaired transmission of information from these proprioceptors to the brain, causing balance issues, sudden jerky movements and misperceived reaction times to the environmental surroundings; for example, thinking objects, such as cars especially when in a vehicle, are closer than they actually are. In these cases, driving can become extremely dangerous and caution should be used. If your proprioception interferes with driving a vehicle at all, look for alternate types of transportation until normal proprioception has returned.

I know this may sound impossible, but better it be possible than fatal. We all notice "bad" drivers making risky unsafe moves. Let's imagine an unsafe move in front of a proprioception challenged individual; not a pleasant thought! Think safety first. Your loved ones will thank you even without words. For those of us who get to be driven around town as if we were "Miss Daisy", when experiencing those proprioception difficulties, just pull the sun visor down in the car to block out some scenery from your viewpoint, wear sunglasses and look down or away if needed. You may feel like you're in a go-cart or a bumper car, but in between jumping like you're going to hit, try to relax.

Think, "There's no place like home, there's no place like home." You will eventually get to your destination and may even want to kiss the ground thinking, "Whew, I made it! Thank you, Lord! Praise God!"

Proprioception can be improved by certain exercises for instance, with a balance or wobble board or even a Bosu ball. Balance and wobble boards work by allowing your body to help make those connections in the brain by improving the feedback between your sensory nervous system and the brain with repetitious movements. Rehabilitation by using balance and wobble boards is available through both physical therapies that specialize in concussions and by good physiotherapists. Wobble boards can be purchased for home use practice as well online and in retail fitness sections.

Exercises start from a sitting position with feet placed on board making alternating movements from front to back, side to side, and circular motions of clockwise and counter clockwise. Exercises then proceed to a standing position, but please make sure to do them while holding onto a sturdy object such as a chair or countertop to help with balance; repeating the consecutive movements of motion. After performing these exercises, both sitting and standing while holding on are accomplished fluently, you can then proceed to standing unassisted balancing while accomplishing these exercise movements.

Make sure however that there is something solid to grab a hold of in case if dizziness or vertigo appears, such as a counter top, solid chair, et cetera. If dizziness or vertigo does appear, stop and rest before proceeding. Then restart by going back to the sitting position again, then standing while gripping onto a solid object. Just think, when you get really good at it, you can "wobble" on one leg and amaze your friends. Please use caution as you know your own body. If you have used one in the past but have stopped and are now having some difficulties with proprioception, dust yours off and use it. Sometimes it's just hard for our body to know where we are at in relation to time and space, with all of the bombarding stimuli our brain receives on a daily basis. So let's go ahead and make those sensory brain connections. Besides, it's fun!

Hormonal Imbalance: After a brain injury you're not going crazy, your hormones might just be all out of whack. When we suffer a head injury, there can be damage to the hypothalamus and the pituitary gland (known as the body's "master gland") resulting in pituitary dysfunction, to the extent that the hypothalamus and the pituitary gland may not fully recover. This damage to the pituitary gland can further cause havoc throughout bodily systems and as a result, bring on many symptoms; because all of the endocrine glands are under its control for supplying the body with the exact amount of hormones it needs to function properly.

We may experience a decline in hormones due to the pituitary gland no longer producing the much needed "normal levels" of hormones due to the hypothalamus regulating the hormone production release from the neurological input it receives throughout the body. This leads to compromising the connection to the entire endocrine system, which further causes more distress, including missed and irregular menstrual cycles for women, that can all be quite puzzling if not extremely frustrating.

There can also be an increase in Prolactin levels, a hormone secreted by the pituitary gland that is responsible for ovulation, nursing, menstrual cycle regulation, metabolism, regulation of the immune system and aides in pancreatic development as well. Due to the imbalance in hormonal levels, it poses a strain on the adrenal glands, further compromising your hormonal balance, potentially causing very serious consequences that can ultimately result in adrenal fatigue; which then further affects many systems throughout the body.

There is such meticulous preciseness in the human body when it comes to hormonal levels and the brain's function on the entire body that it should surely challenge anyone believing on a random or evolutionary theory. As this exact precision is critical for optimal health, it undoubtedly points to the intelligent design of a higher power or creator. When there is an imbalance in the human body, then there is a domino effect setting the stage for dysfunction and disease throughout the entire body with all sorts of symptoms taking place that are often misdiagnosed and unexplained by the medical community.

For females, hormonal balance is especially important because when there is an imbalance of the reproductive hormones with an excess of one hormone over the other, as in the case of estrogen dominance from extremely high estrogen levels that can sometimes be caused by damage in the brain, there can be several devastating effects on the body ranging from irregular menstrual cycles with an increase in menstrual flow, clotting, anemia, increased weight with fat stores, fibroid tumors, stroke risk, high blood pressure spikes, cancer risk of both breast and ovarian, and can also trigger autoimmune disorders such as Rheumatoid Arthritis and Fibromyalgia.

When hormonal imbalances resulting from brain injuries cause adrenal compromise and fatigue, the stage is set for disease. That is why it is very important to have blood work drawn after a brain injury and to continue to monitor hormonal levels.

Initially following a brain injury there may be an absence of menstruation immediately followed by an increase of unpredictable menstrual cycles with an increase in menstrual flow and duration as the adrenal glands become stressed due to damage to the hypothalamus and pituitary gland. If there is any evidence of proprioception difficulties or hypervigilance being observed, that means that the body is actually fixed in a constant state of being on alert, further compromising any hormonal balance affecting cortisol levels as well. This is most often noticed in a car with other oncoming traffic or even parked cars but can also be evident when sounds approach from behind.

If the injured individual is extra alert and jumpy to the surroundings, there is then a "fight or flight" response resulting in the adrenal glands pumping out the hormones accordingly to address the presumed stress. Therefore, if there is damage to the hypothalamus and the pituitary gland from a brain injury, there is a disconnect as the pituitary gland cannot effectively trigger the Adrenal Cortex to release in the correct amounts the corticosteroid hormones, glucocorticoids and cortisol (Hydrocortisone) which is responsible for converting fats, protein and carbs, as well as cardiovascular function, and regulation of blood pressure. Synergistically Hydrocortisone works with Corticosterone to suppress inflammatory responses and regulate immune responses. The Adrenal Cortex also plays a role in the release of estrogen and testosterone so when there is a disconnection between the adrenals and the pituitary, there will eventually be displayed adrenal fatigue, as the outcome can be an overload of estrogen in the body.

With any brain injury, especially if one is experiencing hypervigilance there is an overall increase in the stress response as the Sympathetic Nervous System is engaged under the stress. The Adrenal Medulla secretes Epinephrine to increase blood sugar levels and heart rate, Norepinephrine is then released causing vasoconstriction and high blood pressure; which can also therefore have a negative effect on Post-Concussion Syndrome symptoms by increasing them. The increased stress response is known as "storming" and can present an otherwise seemingly peaceful individual as being in an extreme or chaotic state within their bodily systems.

Also observed along with the spike in blood pressure to extremely high systolic and diastolic levels to seemingly display a hypertensive state in an otherwise healthy blood pressure individual, are an increase in temperature, respiration, pulse and an altered level of consciousness. There may also be a decline in human growth hormone (HGH) which serves as being a neuroprotective as it promotes the regeneration of nerve tissue. Therefore, the deficiency has been associated with cognitive decline and memory loss which may be persistently ongoing long after the injury.

Having a complete hormonal blood work profile drawn that includes reproductive hormones as well as DHEA levels either by a physician or gynecologist, then seeing an endocrinologist if hormonal values are out of range at all or unbalanced in any way, will help not only with recovery but with overall health and homeostasis. DHEA (Dehydroepiandrosterone) is a steroidal precursor hormone produced by the adrenal glands that not only serves to fight against aging and disease processes in the body but is also associated with protecting brain tissue under such conditions as stroke and trauma damage that occur to the brain.

Self-prescribing by predicting the milligrams of DHEA dosage however is difficult as one's hormonal levels may vary and a heightened increase of DHEA in the system could offset other hormonal values such as estrogens, which could further disrupt homeostasis. Therefore, it is best to take DHEA under medical supervision prescribed by a physician as some higher milligram value supplements that are sold over-the-counter may be too high for your body's optimal health and could end up being harmful.

There needs to be a perfect balance when it comes to hormonal levels in the body so it's best to see a specialist trained in maintaining a healthy hormone balance. Some endocrinologists specialize in adrenal fatigue and reproductive hormones. They are better able to accurately assess your symptoms in relation to the pituitary gland (if it has been compromised at all due to injury), and its function with the adrenal glands in order to better help normalize hormonal levels once again, with the administration of the correct dosages of hormonal replacement therapy, preferably bioidentical.

Hormonal imbalances can cause a number of psychological, physiological, and physical symptoms which sometimes include loss of libido, depression, angry outbursts, anxiety, mood swings, memory loss, inability to concentrate, learning difficulties, insomnia, increased risk for heart attack and stroke, high blood pressure, diabetes, menstrual irregularities, premature menopause, premature aging, obesity, loss of lean body mass, muscular weakness and much more.

The hormone Progesterone (which can act as a neuroprotective when taken with vitamin D), is not only importantly involved in the menstrual cycle, in the production of sex hormones, but also has benefitting effects on carbohydrate, lipid and protein metabolism and has been found to be helpful in regulating hormonal imbalances especially when taken along with Vitamin D.

Progesterone is found to be a powerful neuroprotective agent as it enhances the survival of damaged nerve cells and promotes the growth of new nerve tissue that shows promise in the treatment of acute brain injury when it is combined with Vitamin D. It is important to note that it is not as neuroprotective by itself if there is a vitamin D deficiency in the body. Progesterone offers a protective and regenerative effect on myelin, the protective coating along the nerve fibers. Additional studies reveal that

Progesterone relieves edema as it reduces the swelling of injured brain tissue as well. An added benefit of Progesterone is the controlling of the excitotoxicity in the brain which can act to lessen seizures that can sometimes accompany a brain injury.

Talk with your doctor extensively to see if Progesterone may be of benefit for you and if the benefits out-way any risks, with a complete medical history, blood testing for current hormonal levels and continued monitoring of hormonal levels. As with any hormonal replacement therapy, remember that bioidentical hormones are best suited for the human body as they are easily recognized and metabolized much the same way as its own naturally produced hormones because of the matching molecular structure. They are not synthetic.

Communication Challenges: When symptoms are heightened, we may notice that our speech is not. We may find that we have trouble communicating as our brains seem to have slowed its pace affecting our speech. We struggle as we search for the right words to convey, as if we are attempting to pull them from some huge file within our head but just cannot seem to find the right ones to speak; when we do, they don't come out right. Our speech can be impaired as we try to say a word correctly, but we get stuck on syllables and may even find that we now stutter. The listener may have a difficult time not only trying to understand what we are attempting to say, but may become uncomfortable as a result, which in turn we often take notice of and as an effect, only seems to further our uncomfortableness which may cause us to want to be even more insular. It can eventually turn into a continuous cycle where the uncomfortableness can start before the attempting communication ever does.

With that being said, if we are careful to notice our uncomfortableness starting, we can help ourselves to try and nip it in the bud; to stop it before it completely isolates us. We have to start with being comfortable with ourselves at every point, especially when it's the toughest, when we're full blown symptomatic. If we can just accept ourselves, where we are at, symptoms included, then that's more than half the battle.

Next if we can believe that others really do have our best interest in mind and that it is possible for them to understand, if only they had some knowledge of what was taking place; even if they don't at that heightened moment. We or someone else can help to educate them on the effects of brain injuries and the multitude of symptoms, mostly hidden, that seem to take over in our lives. We can help by way of just being ourselves. Letting them see us when it's not so pretty, when we're struggling to get through the day, moment by moment. Most importantly, if we know that God has us, through all of this, then we can breathe a little easier through a really tough and uncomfortable situation. If we don't, then we will just be struggling more.

There are some helpful techniques to help us adjust. Having a pen and paper or a little notebook with us can help tremendously as we can write what we are trying so desperately to communicate. We may notice however that our handwriting has changed as well, temporarily as we are symptomatic, to the point of resembling a young child's penmanship. Don't fret too much as this is so common and expected, even though it is beyond frustrating, not to mention a little scary as we seem to be regressing.

Think of it this way, our brains may struggle with all of the incoming information, all of the time, when it is trying to heal, sometimes to the point that it just gets overloaded like a crowded multi-lane freeway with nothing going anywhere. And it takes time to re-route to make sure those important lanes are free for life-saving situations. So, our brain may slow our walk and slow our talk to make sure our organs work properly under the heavy load of all of the bombarding stimuli. As it slows down to heal, we just end up with more "break-time" and challenging new ways to find to communicate; in the end, we will gain such an appreciation for others less fortunate than ourselves.

Lack of Energy: You may have noticed that before an injury, such as in the case of a Traumatic Brain Injury you had lots of energy to perform many activities that included physical, cognitive, and emotional drains throughout every day and many times by multitasking. Now, you wonder if you will get through the day doing just one thing. It's like a bank of energy with only so much that you start the day off with that quickly runs out when drawn upon.

After a brain injury, it takes so much more energy just to deal with cognitive and emotional issues, that you get literally drained over almost nothing. You may notice you have absolutely no reserves left as you reach your limit of overload, your threshold, and are ready for shut-down mode. The extreme fatigue and exhaustion just adds to the emotional state, which may cause reactions of instant crying. It is completely normal as this happens to just about everyone. Please don't think that anything is wrong with you, your body just needs a little more rest. So, take advantage of frequent naps, or at least lie down for a while.

You may need absolute quiet as your head is about to explode from too much stimuli, or some days you may prefer a soothing nature sound such as rain or maybe even gentle, soothing music, softly playing in the background, perhaps even just to have your window open a bit to listen to the sounds of the outside such as a gentle breeze with birds chirping in the background. Whatever works for you on any particular day when you need the rest, just take it and get refreshed. Whatever the day may bring, may you have grace enough for that day.

Then Jesus said, " Come to me, all of you who are weary and carry heavy burdens, and I will give you rest." Matthew 11:28 NLT

I will give thanks to You, for I am fearfully and wonderfully made; Wonderful are Your works, and my soul knows it very well. Psalm 139:14 NASB

2

Nutrition & Supplements

It's very important to get enough proper nutrition in your body, especially when healing from a brain injury. A healthy diet will aide in recovery, so it is essential to eat enough nutritional calories to help your brain to function most efficiently. If we have deficiencies in certain nutrients, we can experience disruptions in our brain functions. Since we may experience memory difficulties with a brain injury, it may cause us to forget to eat, or we may just not feel those hunger signals due to the injury. We can set alarms to remind us to eat several small meals or snacks throughout the day, approximately every three or four hours. Also since we may be more sedentary due to the injury, we are more prone to gaining weight, so it is best that the meals and snacks are healthy and balanced nutrition; remembering to eat fresh fruits and vegetables, meats, fish and wholegrains.

Taking multivitamins or supplements can be wise to help in the area that your diet may be lacking in. Please note that not all vitamins and supplements are the same as far as nutritional content. Some vitamins and supplements actually have fillers or harmful additives, and many are made with soy, which is not only not a healthy source, but also quite harmful and disease producing in the human body. Make sure to read all labels with ingredients listed. I recommend wholeheartedly a wholefood supplement called Moringa-Oleifera, that comes in dried powdered form that you mix with water or add to smoothies. You can even fill your own capsules for the convenience of taking when not at home. Moringa is a medicinal grade, whole food supplement which is 100% bioavailable and enzymatically alive, that is widely used for malnutrition around the world. Bioavailability and enzymatically alive is what you want in a whole food supplement because it offers the utmost in nutritional value, making it easily absorbed into the body with benefits to essentially boost the immune system. Moringa is considered to be the most nutrient dense plant that offers many health benefits with its naturally occurring anti-oxidants, anti-inflammatories, omegas, all essential amino acids, vitamin and mineral content and is available in the freshest and oxidation-free form through Green Virgin Products. Here is a quick link @ http://www.greenvirginproducts.com?aff=112

When it comes to overall health and nutrition, let's not compromise but become knowledgeable to succeed in our health. We are given but one body so let's take good care of it at every stage of life, and especially during healing from injuries.

Fluids & Water: Make sure to drink plenty of filtered water as your brain is 75% water. Carry a water bottle around with you as a reminder to drink more water. Dehydration from not drinking enough water can impair brain function, making it difficult to concentrate and may also cause you to feel slower, as it actually affects the brain structure causing shrinkage of brain tissue. Good rule of thumb for how much water to drink is to drink when thirsty, upon exertion (exercise), and to take notice of urine concentration. Look for diluted urine of very light or pale yellow to clear in color.

Note: Some vitamins and medication can enhance the color of urine; check with your doctor for correct amount.

Amino Acids: Amino acids are the building blocks of protein. There are 20 amino acids that the body uses, 9 of which your body cannot make (essentials) and need to be taken in or supplemented.

There is a mix of three branched chain amino acids (BCAAs), leucine, isoleucine, and valine, which are crucial to brain health as they are the precursors of two neurotransmitters; glutamate and gamma-aminobutyric acid (GABA). These neurotransmitters work together to balance brain activity and help it to function normally. Specifically, glutamate excites the neurons and stimulates them to fire while GABA dampens the firing of the brain cells. When a TBI happens, there is damage to the hippocampus, a deep structure within the brain responsible for higher learning and memory. Studies show that an injury to the hippocampus reduces the levels of BCAAs, thus increases the need for replacement of these amino acids.

Amino acids can be found in such foods as lean meat, poultry, seafood, eggs, dairy, plant-based protein sources such as quinoa and lentils.

Omega-3: Omega-3 fatty acids found richly in fish oil are particularly crucial for your brain health. It may even help heal and restore brain function after a Traumatic Brain Injury. Studies also suggest that fish oil or Krill oil can also help slow down age related brain atrophy. Omega-3 fats additionally help fight inflammation throughout the body, including the brain as it helps suppress inflammation after a Traumatic Brain Injury.

Anti-oxidants and probiotics: Probiotics are the beneficial bacteria for your intestinal system, helping to aide in maintaining healthy digestion. Antioxidants help by counteracting any oxidative damage caused by either eating certain foods, the way that they are prepared, the environment and also the stress that is caused by a brain injury.

Turmeric: Another neuroprotective agent is the compound Curcumin that is found in Turmeric, which can help a wide range of neurological disorders including stroke and Traumatic Brain Injuries. Curcumin is also found in curry powder but sometimes in less concentration than straight turmeric. Curcumin plays a potential role in improving Parkinson's and Alzheimer's disease and can also promote brain health in general due to its potent antioxidant and anti-inflammatory properties.

Turmeric is easily found in your fresh produce section, accessible as a root, that can be stored in the refrigerator or freezer until ready to use by just peeling back the skin and cutting or grating a small amount. It can also be purchased in dried powdered form in the organic spice isle. Turmeric can be added to meals, smoothies or as a quick and delicious treat on a spoon, or mixed in a glass of water, along with natural honey, grated ginger and black peppercorn for a natural health boost full of wonderful benefits.

Another bioactive compound found in Turmeric is aromatic-turmerone that can increase neural stem cell growth in the brain by as much as 80%; which then differentiate into neurons and have a function in self-repair in the recovery process.

Gingko Biloba: Gingko Biloba offers improved blood circulation in the body and especially in the brain by increasing blood flow by dilating blood vessels. The herb also improves memory of overall brain function when using it to treat dementia. The Gingko leaves contain flavonoids, which help protect the nerves as well as the heart muscle, blood vessels and retina from damage and also terpenoids which together act as antioxidants inhibiting free radical damage. Gingko Biloba has shown to improve thinking, learning, memory, overall cognitive functions, improving social behavior while reducing feelings of depression, that may sometimes be associated with such an injury as a brain injury.

Celery, Peppers & Carrots: These are all good sources of lutein, a plant compound that reduce inflammation in the brain, which is the primary cause of neurodegeneration, and is also supportive in reducing age related memory loss.

Cruciferous Vegetables, Eggs & Meats: Cruciferous vegetables such as broccoli, cauliflower and brussel sprouts as well as eggs, meats and even legumes are good sources of the nutrient Choline found among the B Complex family, have great health benefits on the brain and may improve learning, cognitive function and memory. They are even said to help in age related memory decline, as well as the brain's vulnerability to toxins during childhood, resulting in protection later in life.

Walnuts: Walnuts are a great source of DHA, a plant-based omega-3 with natural phytosterols and antioxidants which may not only reverse brain aging but also boost brain function and even promote brain healing. DHA is however also found in Krill more plentiful as it is an animal-based omega-3 source.

Blueberries: Blueberries are low in fructose, contain antioxidants and other phytochemicals that have been shown to improve thinking, learning, and memory while reducing neurodegenerative oxidative stress.

Red Meat (Vitamin B12): Since vitamin B12 is so vitally important for healthy brain function, red meat becomes an excellent source of such. With deficiencies in vitamin B12 there is a higher chance of lower scores on cognitive function tests and smaller total brain volume, suggesting that a lack of this vitamin could lead to brain shrinkage. You may even notice an onset of cravings for red meat. Sometimes your body causes you to crave certain foods containing the nutrients you need.

Crab: If you love seafood, you will love the option to eat crab as it contains more than the entire daily requirement of the amino acid phenylalanine which helps to make the neurotransmitter dopamine; the   brain stimulating adrenaline and noradrenaline plus it is a great source of the brain boosting vitamin B12.

Garbanzo Beans & Green Leafy Vegetables (Magnesium): Garbanzo beans are one of the best sources of magnesium besides green leafy vegetables which benefit the brain cell receptors in helping to speed the transmission of messages by relaxing the blood vessels and allowing more blood flow to the brain.

Healthy Fats: Contrary to the "fat" belief of avoiding fats, your body, especially your brain needs "healthy fats" for optimal functioning. These sources can be from avocados, free-range eggs, coconut oils, organic virgin olive oils, nuts such as pecans, macadamia, almonds, walnuts, wild Alaskan salmon, organic raw milk and butter.

Lentils: Lentils are a powerhouse source of nutrition in fighting off depression that can be associated with trauma such as in a head injury. Lentils are packed with vitamin B1, iron, dietary fiber and folate. (Low levels of folate, or folic acid are associated with depression. It is an essential key to the production of DNA and RNA, which is active throughout the brain and central nervous system, effecting the distribution of essential compounds and neurotransmitters). A lack of folate can alter mood states due to the reduction in the production of Serotonin and Dopamine, our mood regulators. Lentils provide 89% of the daily intake of folate.

So, here's to enjoying healthy eating and happy healing.

Beloved, I pray that in all respects you may prosper and be in good health, just as your soul prospers. 3 John 1:2 NASB

Don't be like them, for your Father knows exactly what you need even before you ask him! Matthew 6:8 NLT

3
Therapies

As you embark on the many therapies that may be of help in the healing process of TBI and PCS, it is paramount that your physician refers you to a good neurologist that is experienced with Post-Concussion Syndrome and utilizes a holistic approach to treatment, rather than just prescribe medications that may only mask symptoms and hinder healing by causing more harm than good. Also, it is critical to your healing process to have a complete hormonal blood work evaluation done to determine damage to the hypothalamus and pituitary gland, which should be repeated at certain intervals of every 3-6 months. If there is any indication of hormonal imbalance, please be referred to an endocrinologist to help further determine complete imbalances to establish treatment through diet and bioidentical hormone replacement to rebalance your body. Keep in mind that lifestyle and food choices do have an effect on hormones as well.

Vestibular Rehabilitation Therapy: Dizziness, vertigo, visual disturbances and imbalance issues are quite common following a concussion due to early metabolic changes resulting from the injury; especially if they are not managed promptly and properly, leading to a worsening of symptoms. Vestibular Rehabilitation Therapy can be an effective tool in improving and relieving symptoms due to vestibular disorders, including inner ear imbalance and crystal formation. Vestibular Therapy essentially helps to normalize a person's vestibular response to surrounding stimuli through performing various repeated Vestibular Ocular exercises. Seeing a physical therapist trained in these specific exercises and specializing in neurologic rehabilitation for the treatment of Post-Concussion Syndrome, that also has a solid understanding of all associated disturbances an injured person is dealing with on a daily basis, will be best suited to help the brain injured individual; while being aware that behavioral, cognitive, visual/perceptual, metabolic and autonomic disturbances encompass the entire being of an individual as a whole. Therefore, a specifically trained physical therapist will result in a much better patient-therapist relationship to truly offer help in combating the many disruptive symptoms, which will aid in the overall healing process.

Chiropractic Care: After a Traumatic Brain Injury often-times there may not only be a misalignment along the spinal cord, but also compression of the spinal cord resulting in disturbances of bodily functions by altering neurological function. There is usually an inflammatory response to any compression or damage within the body affecting the soft tissues and muscles, causing pain, and numerous other symptoms. There may also quite possibly be a compression of both nerves and blood vessels that supply the head. Releasing the compression permits the nerve impulses to flow through the spinal cord, releasing and allowing many of the head and neck symptoms to subside. A chiropractor will also help restore mobility to joints that may be restricted from tissue injury, offering pain relief not only for muscles, joints, tendons, ligaments, bones and connective tissue, but for some types of headaches as well. Many times with a Traumatic Brain Injury the person may experience a burning sensation in the head as a type of headache pain, due to the nerves that run alongside the back side of the head, that are also associated with the injury and to any damage or disruption within the tissue and joints. Chiropractic treatments can offer much needed relief.

Chiropractic care is a vital component in recovering from a Traumatic Brain Injury as it helps to reduce the stresses caused by the injury and to also aide in helping the person to find balance in their life during their healing process. Chiropractors can help in the matter of vertebral subluxation, or in terms of the signs and symptoms a person is experiencing, resulting from a dysfunctional biomechanical spinal segment that is fixated. Since the dysfunction actively alters neurological function, it is also believed to lead to neuromusculoskeletal and visceral disorders. Chiropractic adjustment treatments are absolutely paramount in aiding a person during healing.

Chiropractic Neurology: After a brain injury in the form of a concussion, there is damage to the neuroplasticity of the brain which alters normal synapses, or signals and patterns that make up the circuitry of the brain. This results in the many symptoms experienced by a brain injured individual.

Symptoms experienced with Post-Concussion Syndrome are difficulties controlling emotions, mood, thoughts, concentration and processing information as everything becomes much slower and harder to retrieve the necessary and correct words in order to be able to communicate effectively. Other symptoms include headaches with occasional migraines, dizziness, vertigo, fatigue, blurry and sometimes double vision, difficulty tracking objects, proprioception problems, memory issues and confusion.

Through Chiropractic Functional Neurology it is possible to locate the dysfunctional regions of the brain and retrain them in a sense at the appropriate pattern and signal frequencies, which then allow the brain to remember and reform normal connections that were essentially lost due to injury. The reconnecting of these synapses allow the signaling in the brain to occur and the processing to speed up, further allowing a person to feel, think, see and function much more clearly and efficiently.

KST Koren Specific Technique: Koren Specific Technique is a branch of chiropractic therapy sometimes considered to be experimental as it is a form of natural healing. The technique uses an analysis healing protocol to locate, correct and release areas of blockage, distortion, interference, stagnation, subluxation (partial dislocation of a joint), and other stressors in the nerve, mind and body connection caused by distortions in the spine and structural system, to help both physically and emotionally. Therapy is offered through evaluation by use of both hands and the ArthroStim, an electrical device to help assess and make the necessary adjustments. KST is used to improve bodily function, promote healing; to release both emotional and physical stresses.

Biofeedback/Neurofeedback: Both Biofeedback and EEG (Electroencephalography) Neurofeedback have been documented as being successful treatments for Mild Traumatic Brain Injuries. EEG Neurofeedback has been shown to be effective in treating auditory and memory problems associated with TBI's. Through Neurofeedback the brain waves are monitored on a computer in real time and the information can then be used to produce changes in brainwave activity. When deviations in the normal brain activity occur, a computer sends out an audio or visual cue as an alert and are then received by the brain, which then subconsciously adjusts itself back to a normal pattern of activity. With repetition of this process, the brain is said to stay within its normal ranges, decreasing irregular brain activity and the associated disruptive symptoms.

Biofeedback is the use of sensitive instruments capable of measuring physical responses in the body and in a sense, feed them back to the brain to better help a person alter their body's responses. The feedback is visible and audible on a computer screen. There are different forms of biofeedback options available ranging from Heart Rate Variability and Temperature Biofeedback for cardiovascular and blood flow conditions, to Electrodermal Response for the "fight-or-flight" response that is often associated with a traumatic event. Others include Electromyographic (EMG) for pain associated with head, neck, jaw and muscle tension.

Pneumographic Biofeedback which measures abdominal breathing to help improve a relaxation response. Sensorimotor Rythym Training (SMR) is used to learn to suppress certain brain wave frequencies that may measure too high, ultimately causing symptoms or disruptions, and to allow other waves to increase in order to minimize symptoms to be able to regain focus and a sense of normalcy.

Speech Therapy: Communication can become a huge concern especially if your symptoms include slowed and slurred speech. It is both troubling and disheartening because while being symptomatic with these particular symptoms, the individual is usually highly aware of just how they are trying to communicate, so it becomes absolutely frustrating. We hear ourselves trying to talk in a very slow manner with a slur that can make the listener quite uncomfortable; even sometimes judgmental as they may be quick to judge how we became that way, if they do not know our story. At a first impression, the listener may think that the individual is intoxicated, especially if an unbalanced gait is present. Through educating the public on the damaging effects of brain injuries, hopefully that stigma will soon change.

Speech Therapy can be helpful in ways by both minimizing the anxiety that so often accompanies such symptoms and by introducing useful techniques to navigate through each person's own unique and individualized need for communication. A good speech therapist will patiently go over pronunciations of words, grow or re-grow a vocabulary to both recognize words, pair them with pictures for recognition and help one's speech become more fluent, while introducing memory therapy as well.

Difficulties with speech may be temporary or even sometimes permanent in a sense that it becomes pronounced during heightened and frequent stimuli. It can become difficult both for the injured individual and also for others who may be trying to communicate as well. Please be patient with yourself and others as you recover. It is a learning process as well as a healing process. Alternate communication such as writing down the words you are trying to convey is another great way to communicate, especially if your speech becomes challenging.

There are many, many therapies available to try; find out what may work best for you. Everyone has a specialty, a gift, something they are good at in the way of helping others. Select people are trained in therapeutic ways that can really help individuals going through tough times and especially resulting from injuries and the effects they have on us, on so many levels. Take every opportunity to explore what may be beneficial for you. May the Lord lead you to the perfect therapy on your road to recovery.

Call upon Me in the day of trouble; I shall rescue you, and you will honor Me. Psalm 50:15 NASB

Let us therefore come boldly unto the throne of grace, that we may obtain mercy, and find grace to help in time of need. Hebrews 4:16 KJV

4

<u>Sound & Noise Intolerance</u>

Oftentimes after a head injury there will be noise intolerances, because certain pitches and frequencies of sound can disturb you so immensely as to bring about immediate symptoms. It is a common complaint with individuals suffering from a Traumatic Brain Injury as there is an intense hypersensitivity to sound, called hyperacusis. The auditory system becomes very sensitive to external environmental noises of many sources. The sounds can be anything from people talking (chatter), dishes clanging, certain musical instruments such as violins and guitars, to even children's higher pitched voices. One moment you can feel fine and on the way to recovery, the next moment due to a particular sound, your symptomatic again and suddenly unable to function.

It is very disheartening and frustrating as you may feel like you can't even be around anyone or anything, as there is a complete overload in your head that your brain is just unable to filter out as it once did. Places of such disturbances often include: schools, work, restaurants, friend or family gatherings and concerts, to name a few. But don't worry. There are simple little ways to help combat this distress and make it a little more manageable, so just hang in there.

Sound Meter Apps: If you have a smart phone or device you are going to be happy because there are free app downloads available to measure sound frequencies in any environment you may find yourself in. It will monitor the frequencies even as they change; this way you will learn just what frequencies are problematic and symptom causing little stressors. These apps are available through the app or play store on your phone or smart device.

Ear Plugs: No, not those foam ones that block everything out, so you feel like a zombie and just smile with a wave, because you have no clue what anybody is even saying anyway. I'm talking about the high-fidelity ear plugs. They are these unique, professional grade ear plugs that musicians use, that still allow you to be part of the fun, and actually hear what someone is saying, all while blocking out those annoying and very troubling decibels.

Wow, what an invention! You can look for these high-fidelity ear plugs online; make sure to you view the rating for each set. Purchase ones with a noise reduction rating of at least 12 decibels; some are even rated between 18-24dB. Also available are custom fitted earplugs that are essentially noise dampening ear filters called ER 15/25 that are available through an audiologist. Studies show that ear filters can reduce overstimulation, or massive sensory excitation, to the auditory system caused by various sounds which allow a person to once again participate in social situations without becoming completely overwhelmed.

Quiet Room to Recover: This little oasis can be anywhere, as you will know it once you find it. You will have that "awe" moment of calm, and your brain will thank you. It can be a quiet bedroom, bathroom, or even the car, if that's the only quiet spot; "Hey, whatever works". There is no correct spot, just whatever is perfect for you at the time. Take at least a few moments, up to however long you need to recover a bit from your brain being overwhelmed or bombarded with stimuli. As you relax, concentrate on your breathing, taking in slow deep breaths and release them just as slowly, trying counts of 4-5 of each inhale and exhale. Then breathe normally again as you find your symptoms easing up. When you are better able to return to the activities at hand, just pace yourself. Get to know your limits. If you start to feel symptomatic again, just return to your little oasis.

Quiet moments are moments to be treasured for sure, now more than ever. Learn to accept these times as moments in your life that allow you the time to just let your mind shut down, to let go of all the bombarding thoughts and stimuli that are invading your brain, to just have that "nothingness" for a few moments; true quiet down time.

If you happen to notice that you are able to handle soft sounds, you may find that relaxing outside, or indoors with a window open, weather depending of course, can offer a soothing atmosphere if you are able to hear nature sounds quietly. However, if your surroundings do not offer such, through the technology of computers or smart phones you can quickly pull up some pleasant and tranquil sounds that may bring a relaxing environment to you as you let the symptoms just fade away or at least lessen to some degree. Searching online for soft soothing sounds can encompass nature, water, or even ultra-slow and quiet music; whatever offers a comforting and relaxing atmosphere. Find what best helps you as you graciously accept your quiet moments as a time that your body truly does need. In the process, may you find peace amongst the chaos. Quiet moments are the moments when God whispers, as the world is loud.

And the LORD spoke to you from the heart of the fire. You heard the sound of his words but didn't see his form; there was only a voice. Deuteronomy 4:12 NLT

Also I heard the voice of the Lord, saying, "Whom shall I send, and who will go for us? Then said I, "Here am I; send me." Isaiah 6:8 KJV

5

<u>Sight & Light Intolerance</u>

Certain wave lengths of light can disrupt or alter your vision after a head injury. Particular light fixtures such as fluorescent lighting, can be a huge culprit to bring on disturbances and headache symptoms. Blurriness, blind spots and double vision sometimes plague injured individuals as well. It is best to have an eye exam by a behavioral optometrist or doctor, belonging to the NeuroOptometric Rehabilitation Association who can perform a comprehensive vision evaluation. Their experience can rule out other predisposing health concerns to effectively determine the best course of action for your own unique needs. At the very least, be sure to let your eye doctor know about your brain injury, the symptoms that you are experiencing and how they are triggered. If your doctor is not well versed on visions problems resulting from brain injuries, ask for a referral to an eye specialist who is.

With most brain injured individuals, the energy once used by the brain to filter out irrelevant and unnecessary visual information is now diverted to basic functions of the body, causing an overwhelming feeling from just too much information in the form of visual stimuli to decipher. Remember, visual problems can have a compounding effect with cognitive deficits as well, further adding to the symptoms being experienced.

Glasses: Prism glasses are meant for those suffering from double vision. Occasionally as a result of a brain injury, the vision can be affected in such a way that the person may see a double image. It happens when the image that one eye sees is not in line with what the other eye sees; creating an impression of two images, or a double image. Prism glasses are used to help correct the misalignment.

Tinted prescription eye glasses as well as polarized tinted sun glasses can block out brightness and certain wave lengths of light that can cause a disturbance which could lead to the onset of symptoms.   Prescription glasses can also be designed to block out glare that is often caused by sunlight reflecting off of various surfaces, including water, windows and white colored objects, resulting in an uncontrolled brightness.

There is also specially designed eyewear available that are precision tinted with colored overlays on the lenses that help filter bothersome pulsations of light, that is common in computer screens and other light sources, which have what is called, Spectral Filters. These specially designed precision tinted lenses are for each individual's specific needs. They act as a filter blocking out the exact offensive wave lengths of light that cause extreme stress on the brain and perceptual difficulties from sensitivity to light, glare, contrasting bright colors and even patterns which initiate physical, cognitive and emotional disruptions.   These individually designed glasses with colored overlays, lenses, and filters are known as the Irlen Method and is said to improve the ability to function by reducing and possibly eliminating perceptual disturbances. The glasses are designed to allow the brain to function more normally, to help it heal as the colored lenses calm the brain and reduce stress on the central nervous system. Here is the contact information on these lenses: http://irlen.com/howthe-irlen-method-helps-the-effects-of-head-injuries/

Hat or Sun Visor: A hat or a sun visor can narrow your vision field above your eyes helping to block bright light from shining down into your eyes that may cause a disturbance and possibly act as a precursor for symptoms. Likewise, a car visor helps by blocking extra light as well as additional visual stimuli.

Avoid Fluorescent Lighting: Fluorescent lighting has long been an offender of brain injured individuals by stimulating the onset of symptoms. They may be difficult to avoid however as they are widely used in many public buildings, including workplaces, schools and stores; not to mention some computer screens. Due to the onset of the heightened sensitivity to light, fluorescent lighting can be one of the most disturbing due to the increased pulsations of light within the bulbs that your brain notices, disrupting your body's functioning and producing instant headaches, once the light hits your eyes. If at all possible, avoid fluorescent lighting, even by simply turning the light off. It is the simplest way to avoid it. If however, that is just not possible, then replace fluorescent bulbs with incandescent lighting as the warmer yellow or orange colors are more soothing and relaxing; less bothersome and disturbing.

Computer Monitors & LCD TV's: Computer screens or monitors, whether in the form of stand-alone monitors, laptops, or even smart devices, can cause visual stress on the eyes resulting in symptoms ranging from headaches, (some of which are migraines, some vestibular in origin causing an imbalance with dizziness and vertigo, as well as tension type), to fatigue, nausea, overall discomfort, glare and light sensitivity.

There is a constant flicker of approximately 30 HZ which allows the screen to consistently update new information with the lighting on such devices; some of which are due to fluorescent tube back lighting LCD's (Liquid Crystal Display) which although use less energy, is either made with an active or passive matrix display grid and conductors that allow current to flow through in order to light the pixels. The difference is, the newer active matrix LCD's contain a transistor which allows for less current to control the lighting of the pixels, to give sharper images. With some of the passive matrix LCD's, there is dual scanning where the current scans through twice within the same amount of time, possibly causing more flicker.

With LCD monitors, the flicker or temporal distortion is mostly unnoticeable except in some cases with a brain injury as it becomes a visual stimuli overload peripherally due to the rod cells being grouped in the peripheral vision. Some monitors that are said to be flicker free actually use what is called Pulse Width Modulation or PWM, a method to reduce the perceived luminance of the screen by cycling the light off and on very rapidly at a frequency mostly unnoticed by the naked eye.

However, the brain still perceives the flicker with brain injured individuals and that can be very disturbing as well as symptom inducing. PVM has been used for dimming the backlighting and may be noticeable at lower brightness settings resulting in a worsening of flickering if the brightness is lowered, enhancing the bothersome symptoms. The flicker from LED (Light Emitting Diode) monitors may be even more noticeable because LED's are able to switch on and off even faster.

So, what is one to do? You can either upgrade your display or purchase a computer screen overlay (yellow and orange are most soothing), which is also available from the Irlen Syndrome Foundation with a link below. There are also apps available to change the lighting on your computer to a more natural form of lighting that is less bothersome. Below are additional helpful links to change the lighting on your computer screen, available eyewear lenses to help combat fluorescent flicker, and also a flicker free monitor database to help you in your search for a true tested flicker free monitor.

https://justgetflux.com/
https://www.theraspecs.com/why-theraspecs/
http://irlen.mybigcommerce.com/colored-overlay-clingsfor-computers-tablets-phones/

http://www.tftcentral.co.uk/articles/flicker_free_database.htm

Until you are able to get a true flicker free monitor that offers a non-flickering dim light or a colored overlay to place on top of your computer screen, there are other ways to help combat the symptom inducing bright light flicker monitor syndrome, pun intended, other than not being on a computer and viewing a screen at all, because sometimes we just need to. Try to minimize any external glare, take frequent breaks (For instance, follow the 20/20 rule. Every 20 minutes look at something 20 feet away for 20 seconds), use larger text, use softer lighting in the room with yellow and orange hues, wear precision tinted eyewear specially designed to help filter out the bothersome pulsations of light from computer screens, and blink frequently. Remember that computer screens visually emit blue wavelengths of light that can often be disruptive visually so experiment with what works best for you and don't give up. You will find something that helps as you just persevere.

Window Films to Block Glare: This is such a great little solution to the highly offensive and headache producing glare on home windows; I only wish I realized this earlier rather than 2 years into my recovery. They are reasonably priced and come in many decorative designs from opaque to the faux stained glass look which are quite pretty. They end up enhancing your home to the point of offering such beauty or elegance that you may even wonder why you haven't placed them on some windows sooner. They work perfectly by blocking out that bright glare, especially if sunlight frequently reflects off of anything white nearby, such as another white building or home. They let in a diffused light that still brightens up the room as the design of the window film leaves a tranquil atmosphere. I just love mine! They are available at home centers and online.

Your eye is a lamp that provides light for your body. When your eye is good, your whole body is filled with light. Matthew 6:22 NLT

For we walk by faith, not by sight. 2 Corinthians 5:7 NASB

6

<u>Memory Lapses</u>

When doing the once thought to be normal tasks of our daily living such as cooking, laundry, cleaning, driving, working, and any other chore or responsibility that we seemingly take for granted, we may now suddenly realize that they require much more effort to accomplish both in remembering how, and in the energy needed to accomplish them. We can be left with more than a feeling of being on a spiraling ride of confusion as to why, but also with a sense of helplessness.

A simple task that we may have always done without even thinking, that is to say, giving any conscious thought to it whatsoever, is now something we need to re-learn. Then remember all of the steps necessary to fully carry them out. We also now seem to need reminders of what it is we are even doing at any given moment, and how to do it in the first place. It is almost as if we have never done it before. Past experiences become more of an echo rather than a memory.

It's this craziness that brings about emotionally charged confusion, and maybe even some guilt for no longer knowing these simple, yet complex tasks. We find ourselves searching for help among a dazed maze we are trying to navigate through, wondering if we will ever be normal again. We hope and pray that we won't forget something too important, like the kids, or turning off the stove. We gasp at how this can all happen as we at times feel completely capable, but then soon learn quite abruptly of our incapability; that it's all just out of our control. We may even think we are no longer competent or efficient as we once were. So, we cry out a big, "Help!" in search of ways to make life manageable again. Here are a few quick tips to help in keeping track of the important things to remember. Please remember, you are not alone.

Notebook: Keep a notebook nearby, by the phone or on the countertop where you will see it, to keep track of all the things that you would like to remember, even of your symptoms and how certain activities affect you. Have a new page available for each day. You can use it as a memory diary as well that can also include important names, important phone numbers, addresses, dates, et cetera. This may help you to feel a little bit more organized with life and all that it encompasses. You can even place little tabs on select pages for each new week to help ease referring back to needed pages.

Bracelet: A bracelet is a great tool to use as we can place it on our wrist to help jog our memory to a task that we are in the middle of. If you can find an unusual bracelet (or better yet, add a jingle bell to it, this way you can also hear that you are wearing it even if you forget that you are, because that does happen), then you will have an extra aide to help out during your daily activities. The sound of the jingle bell will help you to recognize the importance of your task at hand that you do not want to forget. Having a spot to hang the bracelet nearby when you are done with it is just as important, so it will be convenient to grab as you will be able to visually see it upon the beginning of your task and remember to use it. You could even have several bracelets located at different points or areas of your home, for instance: one for cooking near the stove, one for laundry near the laundry area, et cetera. It's a simple little tool that offers great big help.

Sticky Notes: I'm a big fan of sticky notes, or even just a ripped piece of paper and tape for that matter. I have them all over the house, within reason of course, with reminders of everything from groceries that are needed, to bills that need to be paid, to important reminders of events; even something little that I may just happen think about that I really do not want to forget the following minute, because boy do I forget. Notes are a quick convenient way to help stay grounded and to be a little bit more on top of things. You can even use colored paper; and if you are feeling a little adventurous, you can color code your tasks or reminders.

Calendar: Yep, a calendar, for events, reminders, appointments, bills due, and whatever that needs to be remembered. A great way is to highlight it so your eye can't miss it. The more important it is, the more it can be highlighted. Of course, you can color code your highlighted marks as well.

Alarm Clock: Setting an alarm clock is another great way for those important timed reminders of "to do's", such as alerting you to make that important phone call or pay an important bill, plus reminding you of the time to cook, feed the family and feed the animals (although, they don't mind if you forgot that you had already fed them and feed them again. They just love that and will probably seek out more treats, following you around even more. Then you may think, 'Wow, they really do love me!'). Alarm clocks are perfect if you need to take any medication at a specific time and think that you'll remember like you used too, but don't. I am amazed almost every day when my alarm clock goes off as a reminder of such, that I keep forgetting that I'm supposed to take something at that time. It just blows my mind! No pun intended.

Time really can be a funny thing. It's sometimes very challenging to remember things having to do with time, as it just keeps on moving ahead, while some of us may still feel to be in a specific point in time. I mean, have you ever noticed that the month that you are in does not fully agree with the month that you may "feel" that you're in. I'm always a couple months behind for some reason. I notice this, even though I'm aware and conscious of the month that we're in, yet I still seem to be shocked by it; even more shocked when I notice food expiring as I look at the dates, I think, 'Wow, it's past that, already?' Yep!

Then there are those times when I really seem to have "lost time". I can look at the clock and see the time, then look again noticing that a huge amount of time just seemed to disappear. I think, 'Where did it go?' 'What did I do during that time?' It's very weird and puzzling to say the least.

Using an alarm clock really helps to ground you to the reality of time. Plus, if you have a smart phone or device, they make it real convenient to carry an alarm with you wherever you go, even if it's just into another room of the house.

Memory Games: Anything from crossword and word search puzzles, to copying text such as in a list of items, to visualizing pictures and trying to remember what was in the picture. Anything that makes your brain "think", to make those connections, helps with focus. You can even walk into a room, give a quick visual look round at everything in it, then leave the room and try to remember what you saw by writing the items down on a piece of paper. Sometimes it can be very challenging, occasionally even emotionally charging, so don't be too upset with yourself if it's too difficult; it is okay and you are more than excused.

You may notice that some days will be better than others as well as it all depends on the day and the stimuli that you have been exposed to. For instance, in the case of trying to help your child with homework, like math, it may be just way too much for your brain to decipher and figure out. It can be like, "Wow, it's completely Greek and absolutely unrecognizable!" But, on the bright side you will get to see just how smart your child is as you watch in awe of them accomplishing such a huge task as solving mathematical equations and word problems. If you happen to live in a state that enforces Common Core into their curriculum, I feel your pain as those math problems do not make any sense, even to someone non-challenged with their brain. By the way, if you do not have a child's homework to view, I can send you some of mine; there's always plenty of homework.

But seriously, just pace yourself in all that you do as to not get too overwhelmed. Your brain went through a whole re-routing process with damage throughout. So if we, if you, experience some cognitive and memory difficulties, that is okay. You are still wonderful! And besides, sometimes it can be fun to relearn something again and later to re-gain some of what was lost. You may even find that you now like something that you did not care so much for before. When you do start to notice some improvement, even if it's just little or in small increments, you will notice just how much of a great feeling of accomplishment that is. It really is in the little things of life that matter so much!

Trigger Your Memory: Use a trigger or symbol to remember. No, I'm not talking about those negative "triggers" that send us off into a tail spin and help to cause us to behave in ways we thought weren't even possible, or at least, long gone. These triggers are purposeful triggers to help jog our memory for something that we would like to remember. Ideas can be to place items such as keys in a particular area as to not forget them, leaving the shampoo bottle top open to remind us that we just washed our hair, leaving a light on in a room that we need to go back into to finish something; for instance, laundry. Also, turning your watch over or placing a rubber band on your wrist, leaving something hanging out of your purse or wallet such as a note of reminder, et cetera. They are like leaving little clues around the house or workplace by having something out of place that you will hopefully take notice of, to remind you of what it is that you would like to remember. They are those "Oh yes" moments that we seem to need to function a little more like we used too.

Visualization: For those times when you seem to just have more "brain interruptions" then usual and you can't even remember what certain things or places are called, try to visualize them instead. It ends up being a sort of game, like charades, you know that word association game, but just in real life. Sometimes we just have to give clues to something that we can't quite figure out, because it really has slipped our minds, occasionally to the point of even when we hear the right word for it, it still doesn't even sound familiar; but if we can visualize it, we are half way there. The rest will come somehow and someway. Then you can brush up on your art skills, by drawing what you visualize which can really help with communication. You can also write words that you can't quite speak at the moment. Visualizing paints a picture in our minds and truly does offer help overall with communication.

Repetition: For those short little things you want to remember from phone numbers, grocery list items or something you just want to tell someone, repeating it over and over again in your head will help jog your short-term memory to remember it. You can of course repeat it out loud, then others that hear it can help you remember it too;

that is if their sideways look at you won't interfere, and you end up forgetting altogether. If that does happen, just go back to where you were, it should all come back to you. Repetition is useful, as it does help train your brain in remembering how to perform certain tasks. If you add writing it down on 3x5 cards, it will be a double whammy and can be remembered in your long-term memory by reviewing and repeating daily.

But the Comforter, which is the Holy Ghost, whom the Father will send in my name, he shall teach you all things, and bring all things to your remembrance, whatsoever I have said unto you. Peace I leave with you, my peace I give unto you: not as the world giveth, give I unto you. Let not your heart be troubled, neither let it be afraid. John 14:26-27 KJV

And he said unto Jesus, Lord, remember me when thou comest into thy kingdom. And Jesus said unto him, "Verily I say unto thee, today shalt thou be with me in paradise." Luke 23:42-43 KJV

7

<u>Exercise</u>

As with all exercise you are participating in, please be cautious and listen to your body; get to know it. If you are able to exercise both physically and mentally, be cleared from a medical doctor for exercise, then by all means partake in it at your own pace as there are numerous benefits for your overall health and healing. Exercising engages both the Central and Peripheral Nervous Systems and can reduce inflammation and insulin resistance, stimulate the release of growth factors that directly affect brain cell health and develop new blood vessel growth in the brain by increasing the survival of brain cells. Exercising regularly can both improve and protect your memory, as well as your thinking abilities. It also serves to enhance overall cognitive function, which is increasingly more important the older we get as well as crucial to brain health and recovery from injury.

Remember that you are not competing with anybody else, but just being yourself, doing the best you can for that particular day; and days will differ so please do not be discouraged when you find that you can do much more on one day over another. Exercise can very well bring about symptoms as your brain tries to make those important connections in trying to move and coordinate your body parts while regulating your breathing and temperature during exertion. Paying close attention to the cues your brain and body gives you will help you to better monitor your effort and progress during and after exercise. If exercising is just too much for you at any moment, and especially if you notice any pressure in your head, stop until you are better able too. Remember also that outside temperature plays an important role in how you will feel, especially when it comes to exercising. In extreme heat or on very hot days, you may notice that you become symptomatic much more easily, so bear that in mind and choose cooler days to exercise or exercise in a temperature controlled environment. There is no rush.

Another important thing to remember is that symptoms can compound both throughout the day as well as from day to day. If your body does not get adequate rest, water and nutrients, you are more apt to struggle with exercise and experience the compounding effect. It is not yours or anybody else's fault, it's just what to expect at times.

Keep in mind that heat plays an extremely important role in the outcome of your exercise sessions. If you do choose to exercise when it's hot outside, you will find that due to the added strain of the hotter temperatures taxing the body enough on its own in an effort to cool itself down, by adding another form of stimuli may exasperate symptoms. Sometimes just adding in exercise to the mix, whether your body is already struggling with any outside stimuli such as sights, sounds or heat, can result in really throwing you into a tailspin of extreme symptoms; even though you may have been experiencing less and less symptoms recently. The heat can definitely be a culprit and will bring them on. If it is hot outside and you still would like to participate in exercise, use extra caution if you are outdoors, stay in the shade, plus have someone with you in case you need help to find a place to rest. If you are indoors, have a fan close by. Either way, whenever you exercise be sure to drink extra water. Personally, I would advise to wait for a cooler day as I have personally experienced the extreme of symptoms brought on by heat and it's not pretty. You feel as though you're right back at the start of your injury again. With that being said, here are some tips to help you to gain or even regain some physical fitness, endurance and stamina while you improve your overall health and healing.

Walking: Relearn to walk before running. I'm not trying to be sarcastic or silly with that statement, just realistic. Start off slowly because with a brain injury and depending upon the location of the site of impact, your balance and gait may be off, extremely off where you actually tilt and tip over. That was my experience with walking again as I would both tip and lean to the right. The coordination of just moving my legs while trying to stay stable was a learning experience and a slow process, so much so that I just could never even think of running. However, with practice I got better, holding onto someone at first then trying to walk on my own. You will get better and you will go farther too with practice. Who knows, maybe even run someday, as long as the bouncing doesn't bother your head.

When you begin walking for any distance again, be sure to travel on a flat and solid surface, such as pavement to start. You will find that walking on uneven surfaces such as grass (especially taller grass), leaf covered ground, multi-colored gravel or stone, and even patterned, textured or visually busy flooring, that it will be much more challenging and most likely, symptom inducing. The distortions of the rougher terrain will tax your brain while you attempt to navigate through it. Snow with its brightness and uneven depths will also impose a whole new type of challenging terrain. Walking on these types of surfaces will surely test your proprioception to the max. It may cause vertigo, dizziness, slowness of speech and an unbalanced gait; to the point where you may feel to be in the acute stages of injury once again. If you do however walk on a rougher surface or depth of terrain, make sure to have someone else with you in case your symptoms become too much to handle and compromise your safety.

Please be extra, extra careful and have a person with you who is aware of what to look for in becoming symptomatic, when it comes to walking on any elevated surfaces such as stairs, inclines, and rocky or water areas that could pose an unforeseen danger. Stay clear away from gorges and cliffs for obvious reasons of becoming unsteady and dizzy which would pose a very dangerous situation for all involved.

If you do notice persistent challenges in the area involving your vestibular system and proprioception, seek out further therapy and practice vestibular exercises to help your brain adjust to making new connections and to adapt yourself to your environment; to where you are in space and time.

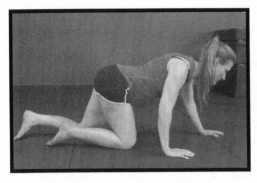

Crawl: "What, crawl?" You might think. Yes! Yes, I know you have been walking and running for most of your life, the very notion of going back to an infantile stage of crawling might sound

completely absurd; because it does sound it. Believe me, just trying to coordinate the alternating movements of arms and legs in a synchronized motion does get very confusing, very quickly and really does challenge your brain to try and make those connections that would otherwise seem to be so simple.

Studies have shown that this movement of "cross-crawling", alternating the left arm with the right leg and vice versa actually activates nerve cells in the brain and stimulates them to create neurological pathways, (synapses) between the left and right sides of the brain. In infants, crawling stimulates brain growth to the point that when infants skip this crucial stage of development, they may end up with various learning difficulties later on including comprehension, speech, reading and writing. So not only is it wise to encourage all children to crawl, even if they just want to get up and walk, but also just about anyone at any age and especially those of us with a brain injury or any cognitive decline and who are able to, in order to help re-create those damaged pathways.

The cognitive benefits of crawling are absolutely priceless as it is a true brain exercise. Try it. When you're finished, you will never look at a baby crawling quite the same way ever again. It's hard. Oh sure, when I started to crawl I thought, 'Ha, I got this!' Well that feeling did not last very long as I was humbled quite quickly. It was really difficult because I was too caught up in which leg or arm to move next that my pace slowed exceedingly, as did my speech again; temporarily though as my brain was figuring out the next move. It really engages your brain to think. Although tough, it can be a real milestone to accomplish the

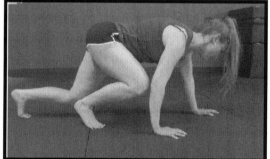

coordinating movements of crawling. It might very well be a good idea to get knee pads or be creative by perhaps attaching a folded sock with a

large enough rubber band to your knees as crawling can be a little hard on them. You could also bear or cat crawl, just elevate your knees and use your feet instead.

Crab Crawling:
"What?" You may be wondering this time, especially if the notion of regular crawling did not engage your inquisitive side. This time we're going to crawl like a crab. Crab

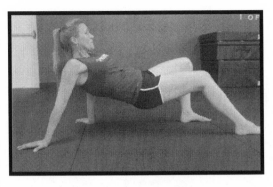

crawling will utilize coordinating movements again just as in regular crawling, but this time you will be facing upright in a supine type of position on all fours while alternating your arm and leg movements. This will be much easier on the knees, (woohoo), as you are utilizing the palms of your hands and your feet. It may feel a bit awkward at first and look quite awkward as well, but the effect is what we are looking for. You will again alternate movements of hands and feet from side to side. You can at first, if it is a little easier, to just move the same side (hand and foot of the same side), then the other side both in a forward motion for a short distance, then continue on to crab crawling in a backwards motion.

Once this movement is comfortable, you can then attempt moving your hand and foot of opposite side, at the same time, to do the same crab crawling motions; and this is where more of a challenge comes into play. It's corny, quirky and can appear to be quite creepy, especially if someone sees you coming towards them, like your dog or cat. So if they get all goofy on you as you practice your coordination movements, beware because the laughter may really throw you off; but it may also make it much more fun.

One-Sided Training: Again, it's that coordination thing and your brain trying to make those new connections with the onset of only utilizing one side of your body at a time; which really does challenge your balance and mobility. It makes you think as you move each body part. It encompasses total concentration for these otherwise seemingly simple, yet challenging movements. First start without any added weight as you adjust to balancing your own body weight. You can start by standing on one foot as you lift up the opposite foot. Hold your arms out to the side to act as a counter balance as you hold still in position. Repeat with your opposite leg until complete balance is maintained.

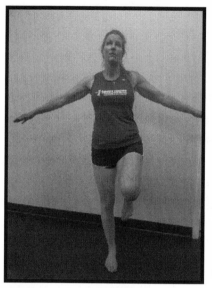

When this position of balance becomes comfortable and easy, you can then try the same while you lean straight forward. Hold onto something stable at first, such as a counter top or chair 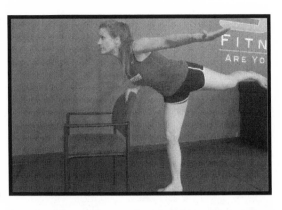 until you are completely balanced and stable with the movement. Next you can attempt this by stretching both arms out to the sides of you, to act as a counter balance, as 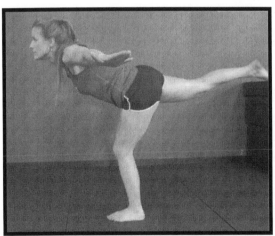 you lean straight out forward, balancing on one leg. Hold these positions as long as you can, working up to 30 seconds, then for 1 full minute. It may look really easy, but it does challenge your balance. When finished, return to a standing position slowly as to not become dizzy. If at any time you become symptomatic, stop, sit and rest. Safety is the most important thing to remember. You will accomplish these in time, but you may need much patience to get there at first.

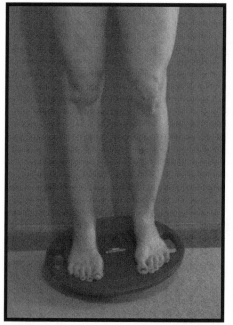

You may have heard of a "wobble board" or Bosu ball and may have even had training since your injury in a rehabilitation setting. They are sold locally and online as well. They really do help with balance as you attempt to shift the weight between both legs to counter any imbalance experienced from the wobbly motion. Be sure to hold onto something stable such as a sturdy chair or countertop in case you become off-balance or dizzy. When you are comfortable enough to try to balance without hanging onto anything but have it close by incase you need it.

If you do not have access to a wobble board, you can try standing on a cushion, but first remove it from off of the couch or chair and place it on the floor; yes, I had to say that. The unevenness of the foam while standing on it will give or flatten in proportion to the amount of

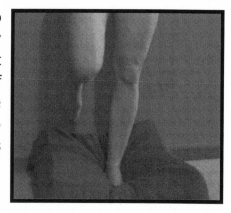

weight applied to it upon standing. You can practice your one-legged balance exercises on the foam starting with just holding one leg up for an amount of time, say, 30 seconds to 1 full minute. Again, for safety, have something stable close by in case you become too off-balance. When finished, be sure to place the cushion back on the appropriate chair or couch, otherwise whoever may sit down on it will surely be in for a surprise. If you really like the idea of standing on a cushion for balance and for help with proprioception, but do not want to stand on your furniture cushions, there are both foam and gel filled balance cushions available online and possibly at fitness or rehabilitation equipment stores locally.

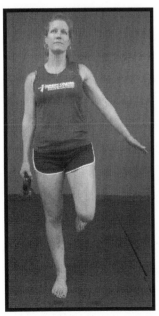

Once you are able to have complete balance, you can then add in weight to the equation which challenges you even more; just not on the wobble board as that would definitely present a danger. Note that by adding weight, your body will try to adjust to the shift of becoming off balance by the particular weight. To begin by adding weight, start with 10lbs. for instance, or less if you need to, on the one side; starting with just standing and walking, then working up to going through a series of movements and flow drills of motion. When you finish working the one side, you can then alternate to work the other side of your body to complete the motions of a one-sided training exercise. It will challenge your balance, your memory, your coordination, and your intellect as it may slow you down mentally as well as physically; temporarily though, as your body tries to make those connections in regaining complete function. It is important to take record of just how far you can get through these exercises until symptoms begin, as the onset starting time of symptoms may increase. That means it will eventually take longer to become symptomatic; yay! Also keep track of how long you are symptomatic for each exercise, as the duration may decrease while you heal.

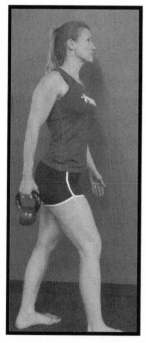

We begin with standing then move onto walking while holding a weight. If 10 lbs. is too much, that's okay, go lighter until you can work up to a heavier weight; it's that "safety first" again. If you do not have access to weights, you can always improvise and use items around your home such as a laundry soap bottle; I'll discuss more on that later on. So, first start by standing with your feet flat on the floor and positioned about a shoulder's width apart to maintain a secure balance, while holding a weight in one hand. If your balance is good, you can try to lift up the same side leg and hold for counts starting with 10 seconds. Then try lifting the opposite leg while holding for the same count. Switch the weight to the opposite arm while repeating the process of lifting up the same side leg, then the opposite leg. Hold for counts starting with 10 seconds, increasing by 10 seconds until you are able to balance for 30 seconds then up to 1 full minute, comfortably and without any balance problems. Again, if you become too off-balance, dizzy or symptomatic, please stop until symptoms disappear. Always watch for head pressure.

Next begin to walk while holding onto a weight in your one hand. As your body flows in the motion of walking you will alternate your leg and arm movements. The added weight will challenge you to re-shift your body to regain and maintain balance as you move. Just like with walking in the beginning post-injury without weights, your brain and body had to work together to coordinate movements in a balanced flow, this too will challenge your brain and your body to do the same. Start by having the weight on the one side of you as you walk forward, then backwards until comfortable. Then switch the weight to the opposite hand and

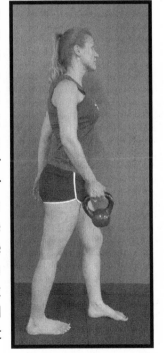

repeat. Remember that safety component? Well it applies here as well.

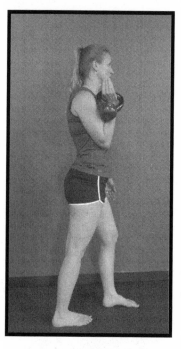

When you have this movement down, if you are able to acquire a kettlebell, you may add another dimension to the walking movements. Place a 10lb. kettlebell in your hand, couched or resting in front of your shoulder as you keep it steady while you walk. It's just another aspect in the one-sided training for walking. If you do not have one, that is fine too. They are however available in stores and my favorite, online. Why is online my favorite you may wonder? It's because you do not have to physically walk into a store and experience the fluorescent lights and face the numerous other stimuli that just slows a person down before they even get started.

Once you are fluent with both standing and walking movements while holding onto an added weight, as long as you do not experience an increased amount of symptoms that impair you, you can begin training with additional movements holding onto the weight. Start with a heaviness of weight that you are comfortable with.

Kettlebell Swing: You can begin to perform a kettlebell swing by standing with a firm foundation over the kettlebell that is placed between your feet while keeping your chest up and maintaining your shoulder placement

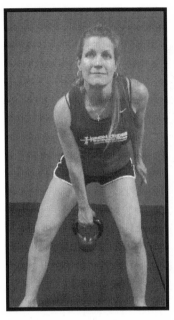

positioned

back and down. You can start with two hands and then when

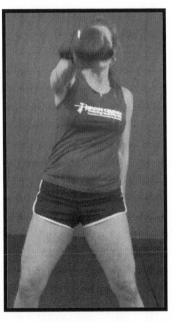

you are comfortable and balanced with the movements, you can perform onehanded kettlebell swings. Start by squatting down and grip the kettlebell with your palms facing you. As you move back into a standing position, tighten abdominals and explode through your hips shifting them in a forward motion while squeezing your buttocks (glutes), to swing the weight in an upward motion, while pushing through your heels. The kettlebell is aimed to be approximately at chest level while your arms, (or arm for one-sided single arm kettlebell swing) are fully extended.

As the kettlebell begins to flow back down and descend, just let the weight flow by gravity between your legs as you maintain your bodyweight shifted back into your heels to work your glutes and hamstrings. If at any point, you become unbalanced or symptomatic, stop and rest to give your brain time to catch up with the movements and exertion placed on the body as it is both physically and mentally challenging.

You are looking for controlled and steady movements; not quick and jerky ones. You are not trying to throw off your balance to the point of injury, (we don't want any more injuries) just adjust or tweak it a bit so your body will learn to compensate. If the weight you are using is causing unbalanced and jerky movements, trade it for a lighter weight. After a few movements, the weight will appear heavier anyway.

If you do not have access to any weights at home, you can always improvise and use a canned good; no glass, just in case and be sure that your hand fits around the can comfortably. You can also use a laundry soap bottle (make sure the cap is tight) for a little more weight. They are actually great because they have handles to hang onto and you can adjust the weight by adding or reducing the amount of fluid inside; and if you're handy or have a handyman around, they can be filled with cement for even more mass. Hey whatever works. They also come in different sizes and you need them anyway for the dreaded laundry that is so easy to forget about; or if we haven't yet, we might like to.

Doorway Push-Ups: For those of us who would love another way to work our upper body (primary muscles used chest and shoulders) to enhance our physique, but traditional push-ups just lend to way too much head pressure as it only ends up serving to bring about those 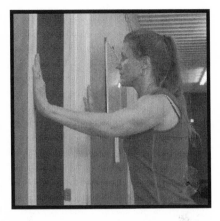 nasty symptoms again, then doorway push-ups are the way to go. They offer an upper body work-out with less strain and pressure in your head. They work the same way as the traditional push-ups except that you are standing upright 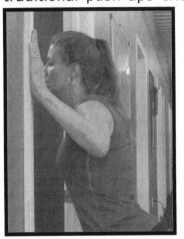 with both feet positioned flat on the floor at shoulders width apart. Make sure to have a stable footing so that you are not off-balance while doing these. Lean into a doorway frame while placing both hands on the frame of the door in the same fashion as you would in a push-up. Example: palms flat, fingers upright at, or slightly above shoulders. Inhale while leaning into frame, exhale while pushing yourself out from the doorway frame. You can start with a series of 10 repetitions and then move onto some creativeness with it.

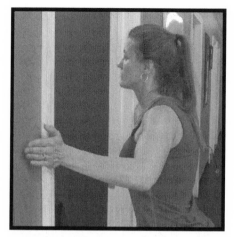

Next, you can turn your hands outward so that your fingers are pointing to the sides of you and arms are a little farther down at mid chest area. This will work your triceps, chest, shoulders and rear deltoids. Repeat the same series of 10 repetitions inhaling on your way into the door frame, exhaling as you push yourself up away from the frame.

When you have that move established and secure, you can really get crazy turn your hands even more, just as long as your wrists do not have any difficulties with mobility or pain, so that your fingers are now pointing downward towards the floor, but with your arms positioned lower towards mid waist. This will present a focus on your biceps, you know, to give you that bump that everyone loves; but this time it's a good bump and nothing to do with the head. Phew!

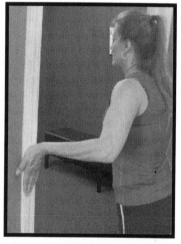

Repeat the same series of 10 reps, inhaling on the way into the door frame, and exhaling as you push your way out from the door frame.

When you are efficient and symptom free, especially regarding dizziness and balance, you can incorporate one sided training into these doorway push-ups as well. To do

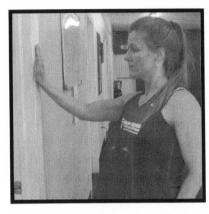

these you would just focus on one arm at a time, to one side of the doorframe at a time. Physically working the one side again can prove to be challenging as before with other one-sided training exercises because balance, coordination and thought goes into each move. These exercises as with the others will again challenge your body, your brain and your brawn. In the end, you will be stronger for them.

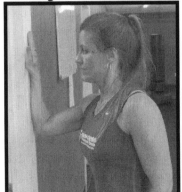

Be mindful of any symptoms should they occur, resting when needed. Always get to know your body and listen to it. If all is good, that's wonderful as you can finally do push-ups again; just a little differently than before, but still quite effective.

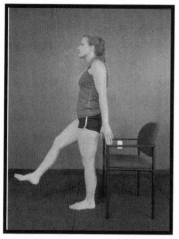

Squats: Yes, those both loved and dreaded squats are available for you to still work them. Okay, so just think of the added benefits of having a natural butt lift. You may not be too concerned with it now, but trust me, when you're older, that would be a treasure of a benefit. We're going to do them but we're just going to do them a bit differently, that's all. First, to make sure and maintain a stable foundation, begin these when you are symptom free and not dizzy. You can begin these by just sitting at the midway point of a chair with arms, while holding onto the sides of the arms with your hands. Have a stable setting for your foot placement where they are again approximately a shoulders width apart in front of you. Begin to stand while focusing on pushing off of your heels as you begin lift

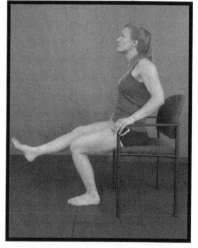

yourself into a full standing position. Your hands will help guide you and give stability if you should become symptomatic. Make sure to stand up slowly as to not cause a drop in your blood pressure, which can lead to dizziness and becoming off-balance for sure. Slow and steady movements are again what is preferred for safety. Perform

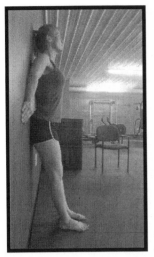

a series of 10 repetitions and see how you feel. If all is good and this is easy for you and you do not experience any troubling symptoms, you are onto the next squat exercise.

Wall Squats: Stand against a wall with your back flat up against it and your feet positioned straight, approximately at shoulders width apart, and flat in front of you far enough so your knees do not go over your feet as you squat down alongside the wall. Let your body just slide down the wall as far as you can

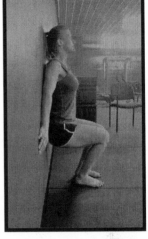

until your bottom is in a straight line with your knees, again paying close attention to your knees not being positioned over your feet. We do not want to add any strain to the knees. Push up and off of your heels again as this will work your bottom and the muscles of the posterior chain. If you can do 5-10 consecutively, but slowly, that will be fantastic. If you can only

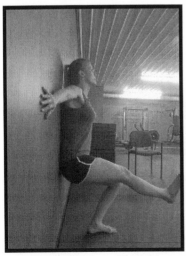

do a couple or a few, that is still great and a wonderful accomplishment! When you feel accomplished and comfortable with wall squats and are really up for a challenge, just try them with one leg and see what you can do; again, push off of your heel as you stand up.

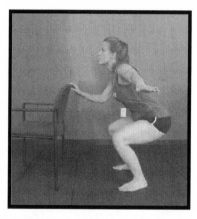

Independent Squats: When you feel completely balanced and are ready to try a regular squat, you should always have something stable close by to help you steady yourself. Again, have a stable foundation for your foot placement making sure they are at least shoulders width or slightly wider apart in front of you. Squat down, being careful not to allow your knees to go over your toes, then begin to stand up while focusing on pushing off of your heels as you begin to lift yourself into a full standing position. Do as many as your body will allow, with slow and controlled movements. If at any point in time you become dizzy or disoriented, take a rest break and resume exercise at a later time.

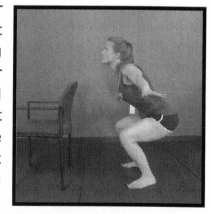

Leg Kickbacks: To help tighten up the back of your legs and give your glutes a huggable squeeze at the same time, we are going to do what is called, leg kickbacks. You can do these holding onto a stable assistant such as a 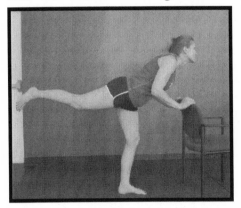 countertop, a sturdy chair, or even the bathroom sink. They are quick, effective and fun to do; plus it will engage your brain as you count in succession. Start with a comfortable number such as 10 repetitions for each leg. Stand with your stable base and foot placement again of approximately a shoulders width apart. Hold onto your stable base of choice. Please make sure no one or nothing of important value or fragility is behind you; trust me, it's really important for reasons I'm sure you can just guess. If all is clear, kick back by lifting one leg straight out and upwards behind you as you squeeze and breathe. We want to engage those bum muscles again called your glutes, and your hamstrings along the back of your legs, by squeezing as we lift. Make sure to breathe during your movements.

As with any exercise, we do not want to blow any gaskets or become dizzy, so breathe. If you can, hold the high position of your leg, at the highest point when you reach your count of 10, while squeezing and breathing for 5 seconds to start. Repeat the same with your opposite leg.

Then work your way for longer counts of repetitions of up to 30, durations of hold to up to 10-15 seconds, when you are able. You can get creative on your own and even hold every other repetition. Whatever will make if fun as long as it's safe.

It is important to note that warming up before exercise with stretching afterward, will help gain flexibility and mobility for better range of motion. It will improve overall conditioning and circulation, while reducing the chances for exercise related injury.

Through exercise movements, warming up and stretching, especially since your body and mind have been through the ringer, it is really important to pay close attention to it in relation to any pain, discomfort or intensity of symptoms produced. Work at your own pace, do only what is comfortable for you. Remember that days will fluctuate as you will find that on some days you can do much more than on others. That is okay. Don't beat yourself up for it! We're just trying to buffet our bodies to help make them stronger, not torture or bruise them in any unhealthy fashion.

If we can start to exercise, even if it's just a little at first, we will ultimately feel so much better, even though going through it may be tough at first, as we may feel just completely whipped. With anything that we practice, we will get better at it. We are built to adapt. You will get better and that feeling will be exchanged for a bit more energy overall. Exercise can and does help to release some of our frustrations and anxious moments that seem to appear out of nowhere. Plus, if we can do some movements outside, even if it's just walking, the fresh air coupled with the beautiful scenery wherever we go will be uplifting and breathtaking; much better than our little enclosed room. You will see that you will gain endurance, feel better and look back one day realizing just how far you've come.

I can remember when I just started trying to walk again after my injury, it was like I was learning to walk all over again. My gate was very shaky with my attempting to coordinate movements and also very limited as my balance and proprioception was way off; as I tilted to the right while I attempted to walk. My whole world just seemed to go to the right. I could only walk a very short distance, holding onto someone mind you so that I would not fall, all while feeling like I was in the middle of a dream state.

This feeling was extremely bizarre. The feeling that I had was that my extremities were not my own; even though I knew that they were. They seemed disconnected from the rest of me somehow. I could look at them, touch them, and try to grab ahold of something with my hands. Yet I was in amazement of the movements which seemed so weird with waving motions and a tingly feeling attached to them, that it just seemed so separate and almost estranged from the rest of me. I remember even questioning if I was awake or maybe asleep and perhaps trying to sleepwalk.

When the feelings of this were intense, I would sit or lie down and rest. When they weren't as bad, I would just keep trying. I was determined to keep going, every day, working my way up to farther and farther distances. So now when I look back to where I was at in my recovery process as compared to where I am at now, I see improvement, big improvement. I know everyone's circumstance is different and everyone heals at their own personal rate. Some are going to have a much more challenging time than others, but if you can see even a glimmer of improvement, that's hope to just keep going forward. Just don't ever, ever give up! You are still you, only a little different, and perhaps even better in a most miraculous way; even if you have not found that out yet.

But those who trust in the LORD will find new strength. They will soar high on wings like eagles. They will run and not grow weary. They will walk and not faint. Isaiah 40:31 NLT

Don't you realize that in a race everyone runs, but only one person gets the prize? So run to win! All athletes are disciplined in their training. They do it to win a prize that will fade away, but we do it for an eternal prize. So I run with purpose in every step. I am not just shadowboxing. I discipline my body like an athlete, training it to do what it should. Otherwise, I fear that after preaching to others I myself might be disqualified. 1 Corinthians 9:24-27 NLT

8

Moods & Emotions

Sometimes our moods and emotions can really have an effect on us; if we let them. A circumstance can suddenly happen which may make us "feel" uncomfortable, especially if we become symptomatic. It can alter our mood from positive to negative in an instant. We may become overly emotional due to the amount of stimuli that our brain is receiving from our surroundings. We may react with anger, fear, confusion, sadness, and even crying; which then might only serve to escalate the situation. We most likely may not even understand what is fully going on, both within our surroundings and within ourselves, but we are for sure experiencing the result of something being completely overwhelming for us.

We do not however have to "stay" in a negative emotion or mood. We do have a choice, we can choose to be content and not anxious. I know that may sound crazy and much easier said than done; after all, our emotions feel real. Right? They are real, but they are not reliable, so in a sense, they very well could be wrong, especially if they are just a reaction to something; like a knee jerk reaction. The emotions may actually be a response to something that our "self" is trying to go into, like a control or protection mode in order to handle a situation. When we have had a head injury, or any other type of injury for that matter, emotional injury included, our body goes into a type of "fight or flight" mode of response. If we are now hypervigilant on top of everything else as well, look out; our body, our "self", is always on the alert to try to protect itself. It can be a roller coaster ride if we let it, but we can decide when it's time to get off that ride.

We can choose to let go of any anger, fear, anxiety, worry, sadness, or any other negative emotion that loves to just have its way with us; especially since we've been weakened a bit by our injury. Let's just turn that around for a moment, looking at it from a new perspective. Let us begin to see our weakness as actually being a strength; a strength that is not of our own. It is through our weakness that we become strong. If you have faith in a higher power, you will know what I am talking about. If not, seek and you will find the strength you need to overcome the negative moods and detrimental emotions that can overpower to take control of you or any of us on this planet. Here are a few ideas to help combat a "bad" mood or a negative emotion.

As previously mentioned in the Nutrition and Supplements section of this book, diet can and does play a role in moods. If we are lacking in a particular area of nutrition, it can be displayed through our moods and emotions. Please refer to that section and research because you may be lacking in any vital nutrients, vitamins or minerals. Remember that old saying that you are what you eat?

Well, it really does hold much truth. So many of our foods are processed junk that contain ingredients, including rotted food and artificial food-like substances that do not hold any nutritional value whatsoever. They are actually quite harmful to our bodies as they are not even meant for human consumption. They are chemical concoctions that are made to look pretty, but at what cost to the consumer! So please take notice of what you eat in the name of proper food as it does have an effect on your body and mood.

Moods: When you are thrown into a "bad" mood or even a down or melancholy mood, try to think about the good things in your life. You can think of all the ways that you have been Blessed, perhaps by a spouse or a love, a close friend or an animal companion, children, talent, career or just that you have had a job, especially because you are still here and alive; that means you're still able to make a difference.

Ponder upon a time in your life where you really felt amazed and thankful. It could be anything, big or small. It really doesn't matter. What matters is to have a thankful heart. How about your favorites and how they make you feel. Think of your favorite color, food, flower, music, movie, quote, or thing to do. Just don't get hung up on not being able to do them at the moment, but think about a time when you will get to do them again. Take a look outside to find beauty in your surroundings, somewhere, anywhere. This is not the end all...it's only, just the beginning.

You can also play some music quietly, if your head will allow. A familiar tune of your liking could be just that thing that brings back a smile. However, you may find that some instruments may not be tolerated well due to the pitches, tones and frequencies. You can experiment to find what works best and most pleasantly for you.

How about a favorite scent such as vanilla, cinnamon, orange, or lavender? Certain smells of scents bring about relaxation and a tranquil mood, that you can simply add to a bath or a diffuser by way of essential oils, or even through perfume sprays. Candles are nice, but I urge extreme caution because when we are challenged with our memory, it is very easy to forget if we have a candle lit. I would advise only to use them when another conscientious adult is home to keep an eye on the candle.

Emotions: Emotions are just emotional, causing us to have feelings and outbursts or reactions to stimuli at any given moment, and then they pass; sometimes just as quickly as they came on. Even though they may "feel" so strong and intense, we really should not rely on them, as they do prove to be, over and over again, unreliable. Anyone can look back at almost any point in their lives and cue in on a particular strong emotion, visibly seeing now that it was essentially all hype. We all get them so we all can relate. With that being said, we should all learn to control them, so they do not control us; in turn sometimes ruin us.

A good way to overcome them before they overtake you is to step back for a moment. Go for a brief walk if you can, even if it's just into another room, such as the bathroom. Think about how you are feeling and what could have triggered it. Ask yourself if it is a valid good emotion that will produce a positive outcome, or a bad negative emotion that could have lasting impressions on more than just yourself; lasting for a very long time. Ask yourself if it's worth it to feel the way that you do? Is it bringing you peace, calmness, real joy or tranquility... or only anxiety, anger, worry, fear, and strife that just settles into your heart? If it is a negative emotion, it is never worth it; even in the heat of the moment.

Now is another good time for those deep breathing exercises mentioned earlier in the book. Start with slow deep breaths of counts of 4-5 during inhaling, then exhaling. As you exhale, imagine that anxiety, that anger, that worry, fear, strife, or anything else negative, just leaving your body. Out it goes, far, far away from you. When you inhale, imagine breathing in love, joy, peace, patience, kindness, goodness, faithfulness, gentleness and self-control. It's a lot to fit into one breath, I know...so break it up. The point is to breathe in the good and breathe out the bad.

Emotions are just a way of our "self" or our pride trying to take control of a situation. It will pass. Remember that other saying that, "This too shall pass"? Well, it will, whatever it is. Try instead to think on things that are good, just, honest, true, pure and lovely; and if you have a higher faith in God, ask Him to help you through. He will give you a peace that truly does surpass all understanding. Your emotions will calm down; you may even wonder what came over you in the first place. You will see the situation in a different light, becoming stronger for having made it through. It's okay, it's all part of being human.

Depression: Depression is said to be an emotional state of a depressed or sad and downcast mood, which is temporary, although going through it seems all encompassing as if it were to be permanent. Many times, in most situations, depression does not accurately fit reality, besides of course in the dealing of a loss, especially of a loved one as the pain is most certainly real. It will not however, last forever as it will lessen. With that fact it is not only wise but best not to make any rash decisions concerning anything of importance, because our frame of mind will change when the depression lifts. When we are down in the dumps with seemingly no hope, with an overabundance of uncertainty, we need to be very careful how we place our next steps, because they could either help make us, or break us.

Our inclination may be to isolate ourselves to just being alone. But that may only serve to worsen the condition, as we tend to dwell on the negative. We may be tempted to take some matters into our own hands, without clearly thinking it over first with a level head of reality, and a true concerning thought for our future. So, in this case it is best to go against our impulsive tendency to be in isolation.

Rather, be with those who love us and want to help us. They may offer words of comfort in just what we truly needed to hear, or a listening ear that does not grow tired, but rather willing to spend the time to really listen to us. Take them up on their offers of companionship, especially when we don't "feel" like it. They can help support us in ways that we may not even consider and in turn help lift our melancholy and depressed moods to let some light shine into our darkness. We will get that glimmer of hope shining through once again. We have people in our lives for a reason; to help us grow, to comfort us, to show us some hope, some love, to help guide us when we're lost, and even to help refine us as if we were a precious metal.

Our down and dreary mood will pass as nothing stays the same. It is but for a moment in time in the bigger picture, even though our present moment may very well feel like an eternity. The sun will shine again. Then who knows, someday, we may be better prepared to help someone else going through the same thing we were. Then we will be better able to give them the comfort that they so desperately need.

Fear: Going through something as traumatic as a brain injury may arouse a bit of fear within us. We may experience a fear of the future for sure; "What it will hold for us now." Other fears may include, "How am I going to pay my bills now that I'm not working?", "How can I keep up with the house chores?", "How can I run my errands when I have a great deal of difficulty trying to even drive?", "How am I going to remember everything?", "How are my family and friends, let alone co-workers or strangers ever going to understand just what I'm going through?", and "How can I keep up when I'm so drained and my head hurts?"

These are just some of the many questions that we may face and in turn create a lot of anxiety, worry and fear within us; which then just makes everything worse. We may become overly focused on us because it is all too overwhelming, because it is really hard to handle, but the negatives will break away once we change our focus to others. All the worrying in the world won't make anything better, not our circumstance, not our relationships, or even how we feel, it will only serve to worsen it. So let's rather just believe, knowing in our heart of hearts that it will all work out. People will help us, our needs will be met, somehow and in some way. Our job or career that we focused on, may have changed a bit, but ultimately for the better; and we never even saw that coming. The house will get clean, when it does; who really cares anyway, you had a brain injury. You're not expected to be "Suzie Homemaker".

Learning to delegate, then hands off is a hard but beneficial approach, which is tough at first because nothing gets done the exact way that you did them, because you're you and nobody else is. Some tasks are done better, a lot are done worse, but it doesn't really matter in the big scheme of things because delegating gives you the opportunity to rest more; that is what's important.

Think of it as they're just learning and eager to please. Others cannot possibly turn into a "you", because they are "them"; not worse, not better, just different. Besides, when your head really hurts, you don't care as much about those things and how the house looks anyway. You just want the pain to stop. So just focus on accepting and relaxing in the moment. Do what you can, when you can. That's it. The rest will come when it needs to. Letting go of being in control of matters is probably the hardest thing to do, but with practice, like anything else, you will get better at it. Don't let the fear of how things will get done rob you of any quiet moment that you are given; or anything else. Be fearless and content with a thankful heart.

Fear is a real emotional feeling, but we don't have to give into it. We do not ever gain anything by worrying about something that may be just beyond our control. If we look back at things in the past that we may have worried about, yet in essence, turned out fine, we then realize that we worried for nothing. When we do worry and get all knotted up inside from the anxiety or stress of it all, it only serves to paralyze us. Then our fear grows and grows. It gets bigger and stronger, as we become fixated on our problems, missing any solutions and blessings coming our way; which can in turn further exasperate our symptoms.

Fear is just a worldly response to circumstances not turning out within our viewpoint of control. It is a "world's view" of how things should be, not true to what they need to be in each of our own unique circumstances. Besides, who is to dictate that view anyway, other people? There is a higher power at work, whether one believes it or not, and things like this are just not in our scope of control. Ever wonder why sometimes the more we try to make things or circumstances be controlled by us, it just backfires? I know firsthand these concerns are very real, like how to afford certain therapies or sessions of treatment due to lack of insurance coverage for them; especially if you can't even pay your bills. It surely is a major concern as an injury to this extent changes your ability to work as you did before. It flips your entire world upside down. You no longer can rely on yourself, your job, or even a family member's employment to be enough for what you need. Your reliance, your focus then changes to that higher power, in a desperate search and longing for answers, to find a strength and a stability once again.

I also know that the more I get to know and trust in God, the more I get to see my needs being met, in ways that I never even factored in. I don't know how or when they will be met, but just at that right moment in time, they are; and that is truly a nice element of surprise.

So, let your flesh scream out in its effort for control as you ignore it, just kick back and make a choice to enjoy the simple things in life, like a smile or a laugh, a piece of chocolate or a delicious cup of tea; whatever your fancy, just as long as it is healthy for you. Just go ahead, enjoy it, noticing your emotions and moods change for the better. Just accept and take the time that you are given in your "down time", to help heal so you can move in a forward motion again. Always be forever grateful as well because you are still here to do just that. Just don't allow worry or fear to drain you anymore. Your needs will be met.

Trust is the key. It may be tough at first if you're like me and have had trust issues in life with people. When unbelief sneaks into the middle of your giant difficulties and challenges that you are now faced with, it can be more than scary and overwhelming; it can be down-right defeating. That's when faith comes in, learning to have faith and trust in a higher power to take care of something as enormous as this. The only One to get us through it all peacefully is God as He is omnipotent (all-powerful, unlimited in authority and power), omnipresent (He is everywhere, all at the same time), and omniscient (all-knowing, aware and fully understanding). He is the One in control; He is able!

We can choose to let go of the worry, the anxiety, and the fear that keeps trying to control us. Just look up and trust the One Who can get us through it all; even all of this. There are several things in life that can induce negative emotions, but few of them are as all-encompassing as an injury of this degree. This is a time that we are facing, and we can't do anything to change that. So, we can either choose to endure it alone, perhaps become bitter and stay a victim, or grab ahold of the One Who knows what we're going through, who can truly help us, so we can become better and much stronger. The choice of which road to travel on is both individually and ultimately each of ours to decide. The question is then, do we want the peace filled and comforting road, or the anxiety and fear filled road.

For God hath not given us the spirit of fear; but of power, and of love, and of a sound mind. 2 Timothy 1:7 KJV

Be anxious for nothing, but in everything, by prayer and supplication with thanksgiving, let your requests be made known to God. And the peace of God, which surpasses all comprehension, will guard your hearts and your minds in Christ Jesus. Finally, brethren, whatever is true, whatever is honorable, whatever is right, whatever is pure, whatever is lovely, whatever is of good repute, if there is any excellence and if anything worthy of praise, dwell on these things. Philippians 4:6-8 NASB

9

<u>Support Groups</u>

Since brain injuries are most often not only misdiagnosed, but also tremendously misunderstood by some healthcare professionals, as well as family and friends alike, they may leave the injured person really feeling like a victim, all alone in their struggle; not knowing or even understanding themselves where they can turn to for help and support. Support and guidance is needed in not only trying to understand the extent of what has happened to an injured individual, but also, with regard to their future in terms of healing physically, emotionally and cognitively; concerning their current abilities and future employment. It can be a real scary time with much at stake in the life of a brain injured individual.

Oftentimes, most unfortunately, symptoms are treated with drugs of both prescription, non-prescriptions, and sometimes street drugs. They are prescribed by some physicians for reasons of lack of knowledge of Traumatic Brain Injuries and Post-Concussion Syndrome so frequently for symptoms that accompany the injury, and for the lack of true compassion for the individual that is injured. Medications are frequently taken by the injured individual both from being prescribed in a desperate attempt to diminish TBI and PCS symptoms, not being fully aware however of the many detrimental side-effects and health risks that they indeed can cause. Injured and suffering persons also may occasionally take street drugs in an effort to numb the pain of loneliness, as this is such a hidden and misunderstood injury.

Symptoms can mimic a severely mentally disabled individual or even one who may be under some form of alcohol or drug influence or in an induced state. A symptomatic person can present with either a frozen or slowed response to stimuli or perhaps even an overactive outburst of response such as abrupt and uncontrolled bouts of crying or laughing at any given moment, while experiencing an unbalanced and crooked gait coupled with slowed and slurred speech. This can become quite apparent and displayed as being way off or not normal. This perceived abnormal behavior can even sometimes be misrepresented as being false or perhaps "faked" by any onlookers. Thus, they are not fully understanding, an otherwise seemingly normal individual, and what they are fully going through due to an injury of this magnitude.

Symptoms are felt and experienced by the injured individual, but not always displayed to others, therefore can be hidden. What is noticed may reflect something quite different, as in the case of an anxiety disorder. Therefore, many physicians are quick to falsely judge the symptoms labelling the individual, as it pertains to a psychological disorder. Then they distribute the pharmaceuticals, which further compromise the health of the individual, rather than just fully examine and learn of the patient. It is extremely disheartening, not to mention frustrating, as the person going through Post-Concussion Syndrome and experiencing the many symptoms can be very smart, well-educated and coherent enough to know what is going on around them, and what is being said about them, but are just unable to communicate effectively. They may be unable to defend themselves, of their condition for reasons being simply due to, overwhelming stimuli. So, an understanding from family, friends, caregivers, and the general public alike is really important and essential for everyone.

Even though the awareness of the complete effects of TBI's and PCS is almost lacking in the medical field currently, there are support groups out there with many people going through the exact same thing; which means that there are people who really do understand. They are patiently willing, and more than able to help throughout the whole healing process, no matter how long it may take.

These groups are available online, through social media, and have many members. They are also available locally; hopefully in your area within a close proximity to you. For the much needed help and concern regarding future employment, there are online sites available that offer links to help ease the burden of the financial stresses that tag along throughout this whole process, through both the Brain Injury Association (look up per state for information and helpful employment links) and Brainline.org., where you can find helpful and useful information regarding current employment and for the future.

There is also a network for job seekers called JAN which stands for Job Accommodation Network, that specializes in resources, accommodations and seeking of employment for people struggling with disabilities. Their website is askjan.org.

BIAA: The Brain Injury Association of America (BIAA), http://www.biausa.org/, offers a network of state affiliates, local chapters and support groups that can help with awareness, education and the increasing of the quality of life, for a brain injured individual as well as supportive care giving for their families.

Locals: Check with your area local doctors, hospitals, schools and churches to inquire about any TBI/PCS support groups with the days and times that are available. The awareness of brain injuries, the lasting effects it has on the individual as well as on their families and life in general, is growing as people are speaking out more, because they are in search of some real answers. People are also becoming more health conscious. They do not want the false fixes of drugs only to mask symptoms, but rather do want to learn more about every possible option available for them, for some hope and real coping mechanisms; if possible, healing.

Some healthcare providers don't always give positive supportive options, either because of their lack of knowledge, or most unfortunately, their alliance and allegiance to the pharmaceutical companies. In which case they may receive "kick-backs" ranging from extravagant meals, pharmaceutical samples, and even great monetary gain for the doctors and their practices. How do I know? I've seen it first-hand working in physician's offices as a nurse, a couple years prior to my injury. I've experienced the lack of knowledge and concern or compassion for patients while I was one, and still am one. So, you may have to ask, or have someone else ask many questions for you.   If you do not receive the answers for the many questions you have, nor the assistance that you need or are looking for, then ask someone else, a second and a third opinion. Keep asking, keep searching; just don't ever give up!

Online Answers: There are many answers online to the many questions that you may have. Some come from a medical perspective offering sound advice and others come from a "survivor's" or individual's perspective offering the emotional side in sharing of the frustration of learning to deal with an onslaught of symptoms that nobody seems to understand; while trying to just navigate through life. Both can prove to be very helpful and comforting as there just may be some invaluable and supportive advice that truly can help. Plus, there are conveniently informative sites that lend important links for specific help and resources that may be directly available to you or a loved one. Some of these helpful sites are as follows:

http://www.biausa.org/,
http://www.traumaticbraininjury.com/injury-resources/tbiimportant-links/,

http://askjan.org

http://www.brainline.org/resources/site_map.php.

http://www.brainline.org/landing_pages/categories/employment.html

There are many more of course with new ones available as awareness grows. But these are a few to get started.

A couple of social media Facebook groups that welcome the sharing of information as members offer support for each other are as follows:

Post-Concussion Syndrome & Traumatic Brain Injury Support

https://www.facebook.com/groups/951850348205135/,

Post-Concussion Syndrome Support   Group https://www.facebook.com/groups/108398302515255/.

When searching for support groups online or on social media, look for positive ones that offer support and comfort from fellow members showing true care and hope, not negative ones that keep you feeling down and depressed as the victim. There are some real negative groups out there that not only serve to keep you down as the forever victim, but unfortunately do not even welcome the sharing of information that can actually help someone; you will know when you find those. Just remember, you're not a victim but a survivor of something traumatic. You can make a positive impact on someone else because of it. These links for groups, as well as others that you will find, are both positive and welcome interaction between members as they encourage the offering of hope and the sharing of ideas. The groups present suggestions that can be greatly beneficial, as well as offering a listening ear as many members help support each other; even if you just need to vent or are in need of a new friend. After all, that's what we're all here for; each other.

He comforts us in all our troubles so that we can comfort others. When they are troubled, we will be able to give them the same comfort God has given us. 2 Corinthians 1:4 NLT

Therefore, encourage one another and build up one another, just as you also are doing. 1 Thessalonians 5:11 NASB

10

Prayer & Meditation

You may have thought. 'Am I ever going to be normal again?' Well, define "normal". By terms of the Merriam Webster dictionary, normal is defined as usual or ordinary (not strange), and mentally and physically healthy.

Let me start by addressing that you are far above usual and ordinary. You are extraordinary; even more so now! You are actually fearfully and wonderfully made! To be mentally and physically healthy, well, look around at everyone you see, we all have something going on whether it's mentally or physically, and that's in all actuality. We are all different in comparison which makes us each unique. We can choose to embrace our differences, our unique specialness, especially now, to be content enough to utilize them to do something positive in life and hopefully help others in the process.

We may also think, 'I used to be this and I used to be that.' You fill in the blank. Example: nurse, pilot, doctor, accountant, truck driver, teacher, personal trainer, chef, clerk, cashier, finance exec., mother, father, student; basically, a functioning human being that knew how to use their brain, but now struggle with even the simple tasks, let alone the thought of finishing in our career, job or school without any difficulty.

So now we may feel that we're left alone to just wander and wonder about what the future may hold for us. We all have these weaker, frustratingly inward negative thoughts because of our unplanned and sudden life change. It is normal because we are human beings just trying to make sense of it all. If we can, let's just begin to take a look outside of our immediate world, and get a glimpse beyond our current circumstance, as it is not forever but just for a moment in time; then our burden of control of our whole situation can start to be lifted.

We don't have to give into the rigidity of a predictable life to just start accepting and appreciating the change every moment by letting each and every one count; even if they're very difficult in the beginning. This is a way to start becoming content with our life and to find joy in the midst of the turmoil. This is life, our life, and it is meant to be explored as we learn to navigate through all sorts of experiences, and take away an appreciation for it. It is all, every moment, a chance to still offer comfort, hope, love and joy to others around us; especially in times when we seem to be hurting the most. The best remedy for our pain is to boldly help someone else; through our pain and through the experience.

Whether we have a hope or a faith in a higher power or not, we will need something more, than just us, to get through this most challenging time in life. I have seen countless times the real difference it makes in a life of somebody injured with such an injury as a Traumatic Brain Injury, when they have faith in God; they actually have real hope in knowing that they are never alone, even through this. They have hope for a future, including a Heaven with a perfectly made whole body and mind again, as well as knowing only God completely understands everything we go through now. As we learn to trust in Him, He will bring people into our lives, into your life, that can help you through it all. In many ways, He will actually weave this whole negative circumstance for a "good", to come out of this! So never give up hope but learn about having faith in Christ Jesus. Try all available resources that are available to you as you may find ones that will really work for you and really help in aiding your whole recovery process.

This type of injury can bring on the absolute most devastatingly debilitating and confusing effects to turn anyone's world completely upside down. It does not respect any particular person with regard to age, sex, financial status, or who we are or where we are in life on the socio-economic scale, or even what we have ever done in life with regard to being a good person or not, but it is sudden and it strikes with a vengeance. Then everything comes to an abrupt complete halt and the effects are not only straining emotionally, physically, and financially, but relationally as well because it will challenge every relationship that you have; and that strain can become ongoing.

This is the time when we learn who we are, who our true friends are, whether family or not, and what we are actually made of as there will be an endurance developing within us.

There may be instances when everyone seems to abandon us, whether for fear, lack of knowledge, or just plain selfishness that we don't fit into their lifestyle anymore. It is the time that at one point or another, we will search for a higher power to just get us through the day and to give us comfort for the moment. That last strand to hold onto as we hit rock bottom and begin to lose all hope not wanting our tears to be in vain.

This injury can be a time in our life when we do find our true friend who is closer than a brother, who will never leave us nor forsake us; ever. One who truly knows and understands what it is exactly that we are going through. One Who will find us the help we so desperately need and bring it to us somehow, someway, even through somebody else.

In the process, we will see these little miracles of us miraculously making it through all of the obstacles that come before us, that would normally defeat us. We will gain endurance to just keep going, even though this can be the toughest and loneliest life event we ever had to deal with as it encompasses everything and tries to conquer us. We will find that we are more than conquerors as we are forged into a person of strength, a warrior having gone through a tough battle, with the help not of our own doing. We will also find that even though we may feel so utterly weak, a Savior's strength is made perfect through us, as He goes before us in all that we face, and we then realize that we were never, ever really alone.

Anytime, throughout our healing process and beyond, we can utilize our time given to meditate on those things which are comforting and pleasant to us; the things that bring a smile upon our faces, even Scripture. We can think of those things which are positive, especially whenever a negative thought sneaks into our mind. This way we can try to lighten our mood, to gain and remain calm. This is also helpful in times of stress related to our circumstance.

We can find a quiet place, take some deep breaths inhaling and exhaling slowly as we concentrate on the things that bring about a calm and relaxing atmosphere. If we can't seem to think of anything at the moment, we can always visualize a soothing stream of water, flowing between beautiful scenery of perhaps our favorite flowers, trees and mountains; a peaceful place full of relaxation. We can imagine ourselves being right there and taking it all in, even remembering some wonderful smells of flowers, grass, pine, et cetera. We can paint that picture in our minds and let the negatives just drift away. We will feel relieved, more relaxed and restful as it should help minimize our symptoms.

This is time of great wonder, although it can be very challenging and emotionally draining. It is absolutely amazing what a brain can and does do. We get to find out first hand just how fearfully and wonderfully made we truly are, as we try to make those new synapse connections between the neurons along the axons that were damaged; to learn to function as a whole person and beginning to live again. Never are we the same again on how we may view things and people, as we gain a whole new perspective in true appreciation of the human body, life, and what's really important. We are struck in such a detrimental way and experience huge overwhelming disappointments with a brain injury.

So instead of becoming negative, resentful, bitter and just plain mean, let us display a sweetness about us that shows others a brightness, a strength, and a hope that so graciously is not of our own but very real and true nonetheless. Let us experience firsthand a crown of beauty for our ashes, joy for our mourning, the garment of praise for our heaviness, to move out of our despair and into rejoicing. Wouldn't you love to do that? Well, you can. Remember that the Lord is always with you, waiting for you, even if you don't yet know Him, or maybe even don't want to know Him yet; perhaps because you're just not ready. There is no time like the present to welcome Him into your life and help you heal from everything; not just your brain injury.

I wish you the best in healing throughout your recovery process. May you gain insight into what truly matters in life and learn a great deal from your experience, both about yourself and others as well. The human body is such an awe-inspiring creation that even through a debilitating or devastating injury or illness, we can still do things like find hope and joy in life every day, appreciate ourselves in what we can do and appreciate others for helping out in what we can't do. Finally, to love others as our heart heals too. Remember that while going through such a trial or season of hardship, the testing of oneself that a brain injury can really produce, you can still learn to endure and gain a strength you never thought possible; all by just finding hope and trusting in God. He sees the big picture past all of our pain. So, with that thought, you can press forward, and you can persevere!

This book would not be possible at all if it wasn't for my faith in Jesus Christ, that through my belief I can see that God truly does have it all, including us, our injuries, and our future. I wholeheartedly believe that there is a purpose for everything that we experience as we are forged and molded to grow in His image; to be what we were created to be. At each step in our journey of life, no matter how difficult or even painful at times, we are gaining endurance and strength along the way if we do not give up but press on forward.

As I look back I realize that He was with me through it all and held me up by His righteous right hand. He continues holding me as He guides me still. He has given me, a brain injured individual, the ability to write this book in the hopes that others will be helped and not give up. Through every weakness I experienced and endured, I was able to add the knowledge and wisdom that I gained and place it into this book. May God Bless you with healing, hope, love, and life everlasting.

To appoint unto them that mourn in Zion, to give unto them beauty for ashes, the oil of joy for mourning, the garment of praise for the spirit of heaviness; that they might be called trees of righteousness, the planting of the LORD, that he might be glorified. Isaiah 61:3 KJV

Therefore, since we have been made right in God's sight by faith, we have peace with God because of what Jesus Christ our Lord has done for us. Because of our faith, Christ has brought us into this place of undeserved privilege where we now stand, and we confidently and joyfully look forward to sharing God's glory. We can rejoice, too, when we run into problems and trials, for we know that they help us develop endurance. And endurance develops strength of character, and character strengthens our confident hope of salvation. And this hope will not lead to disappointment. For we know how dearly God loves us, because he has given us the Holy Spirit to fill our hearts with his love. Romans 5:1-5 NLT

Prayer: Father, when I experience fear, worry or anxiety, help me to cling to Your promise that You will never leave me nor forsake me. Help me to speak and live fearlessly because You are with me. I am never alone. Your promise stands, spoken over and over again in Your Word and satisfying Your followers throughout thousands of years, and continues in this present time.

You are always with me. I commit this truth to my heart right now. May this simple profound truth sustain me today.

In the name of Jesus Christ, Amen.

Afterword

A brain injured person may continue to encounter ongoing challenges within their lives with regard to their health both physically and emotionally speaking as well as cognitively, financially, and in the preserving of various relationships; therefore, disrupting the regular flow of daily living. The continued butterfly effect of consequences in relation to such challenges demand an endurance strong enough and able to withstand each trial. As we encounter these new and seemingly never ending difficult experiences, let us each hold fast to the truth that we are more than conquerors through Christ Who does strengthen us.

Look for additional books coming soon by C. Rae Johnson to help with meeting the needs of individuals with Traumatic Brain Injuries and Post-Concussion Syndrome. Thank you and always have a wonderfully Blessed day through continued hope.

Facebook page- Post Concussion Syndrome & Traumatic Brain Injury Support
https://www.facebook.com/groups/951850348205135/

For Moringa Oleifera:
http://www.greenvirginproducts.com?aff=112

Email: craejohnsonfaithbasedbooks@gmail.com

http://craejohnsonauthor.com/

https://www.facebook.com/Craejohnsonauthor/

http://www.lulu.com/spotlight/CRaeJohnson

'Each time he said, "My grace is all you need. My power works best in weakness." So now I am glad to boast about my weaknesses, so that the power of Christ can work through me.' 2 Corinthians 12:9 NLT

'My soul clings to You; Your right hand upholds me.' Psalm 63:8 NASB

Fear thou not; for I am with thee: be not dismayed; for I am thy God: I will strengthen thee; yea, I will help thee; yea, I will uphold thee with the right hand of my righteousness. Isaiah 41:10 KJV

Notes
Informational Contacts
1-Physical

TBI: Get the Facts, Injury prevention & Control: Traumatic Brain Injury and Concussion, CDC, Center for Disease Control and Prevention, http://www.cdc.gov/traumaticbraininjury/get_the_facts.html

Brain Injury Facts, International Brain Injury Association, http://www.internationalbrain.org/brain-injury-facts/

Da Silva MH, da Rosa EJ, de Carvalho NR, Dobrachinski F, da Rocha JB, Mauriz JL, Gonzalez-Gallego J, Soares FA, Acute brain Damage Induced by Acetaminophen in Mice: effect of Diphenyl Diselenide on Oxidative Stress and Mitochondrial Dysfunction, Pubmed.gov, http://www.ncbi.nlm.nih.gov/pubmed/22081409

Northwestern University, Ibuprofen Verses Acetaminophen For Treatment of Mild Traumatic Brain Injury, Clinicaltrials.gov, https://clinicaltrials.gov/ct2/show/NCT02443142

American Academy of Neurology, Study: Brain Imaging After Mild Head Injury/Concussion Can Show Lesions, https://www.aan.com/PressRoom/Home/PressRelease/1156

Concussion Recovery: Parents Play Important Role, Brain-line Kids, http://www.brainline.org/content/2008/07/concussion-recoveryparents-play-important-role.html

Webmd, Find a Vitamin Supplement, Melatonin,
http://www.webmd.com/vitamins-supplements/ingredientmono-
940melatonin.aspx?activeingredientid=940

Treatment for Vertigo, Imbalance, and Dizziness Due To Vestibular
Dysfunction, http://vestibular.org/understanding-
vestibulardisorder/treatment

Proprioception, Sports Injury Clinic,
http://www.sportsinjuryclinic.net/rehabilitationexercises/lo
wer-leg-ankle-exercises/proprioception

Benefits of Wobble Board Exercises, Sports Injury Clinic,
http://www.sportsinjuryclinic.net/rehabilitationexercises/lo
wer-leg-ankle-exercises/wobble-boardexercises

Proprioception and Balance Exercises, What id Proprioception, Physio
Works, http://physioworks.com.au/treatments-
1/proprioception-balance-exercises

Robert M. Sargis MD PhD, An Overview of the Adrenal Glands Beyond
Fight or Flight
http://www.endocrineweb.com/endocrinology/overviewadr
enal-glands

Denise M. Lemke, Riding Out the Storm: Sympathetic Storming After
Traumatic Brain Injury, Medscape.
http://www.medscape.com/viewarticle/469858

Joseph Carrington, Using Hormones to Heal Traumatic Brain Injury, Life
Extension Magazine,

http://www.lifeextension.com/magazine/2012/1/usinghor
mones-heal-traumatic-brain-injuries/page-02

Donald G Stein PhD, Milos M Cekic PhD, Progesterone and Vitamin D
Hormone For Treatment of Traumatic Brain Injury in the Aged, NCBI,
http://www.ncbi.nlm.nih.gov/pmc/articles/PMC3740793/

Jing Wei, Guo-min Xiao, The Neuroprotective Effects of Progesterone on
Traumatic Brain Injury: Current Status and Future Prospects,
http://www.ncbi.nlm.nih.gov/pmc/articles/PMC3854945/

Carol Peterson, RPH, CNP, Hormones and Traumatic Brain Injury,
Women's International Pharmacy,
https://www.womensinternational.com/newsletter/article
braininjury.html

Am J Obstet Gynecol, 1982 Mar 15;142(6 Pt 2):735-8. Metabolic Effects of
Progesterone, Pub Med.Gov.
http://www.ncbi.nlm.nih.gov/pubmed/7039319

Dr. Mercola, Can this Natural Hormone Actually Heal Brain Injuries and
Strokes? Mercola.com,
http://articles.mercola.com/sites/articles/archive/2009/12/
26/This-Natural-Hormone-Can-Help-Heal-Your-Brain-
Injury.aspx

Prolactin, Wiki, Wikipedia,
https://en.wikipedia.org/wiki/Prolactin

Niederland T, Makovi H, Gal V, Andreka B, Abraham CS, Kovacs J,
Abnormalities of pituitary gland function after traumatic brain injury in
children, Pubmed,
http://www.ncbi.nlm.nih.gov/pubmed/17263675

Joanna Goldberg, Tim Jewell, Medical Review by Alan Carter, Prolactin Level Test, Healthline,
http://www.healthline.com/health/prolactin#Overview1

Head Injuries and Pituitary Dysfunction- Are We Failing to Diagnose it? The International Hormone Society,
http://intlhormonesociety.org/index.php?option=com_content&task=view&id=59&Itemid=1

Heal Traumatic Brain Injury with Bioidentical Hormones, Life Extension Magazine,
http://www.lifeextension.com/magazine/2015/2/healtraumatic-brain-injury-with-bioidentical-hormones/page-01

DHEA Reduces Inflammation Enhances Immunity, Protects Arteries and the Brain, http://www.encognitive.com/node/12840

2-Nutrition & Supplements

Dehydration Affects Brain Structure and Function in Healthy Adolescents, **Hum Brain Mapp.** 2011 Jan;32(1):71-9. doi: 10.1002/hbm.20999. PubMed.gov.,
http://www.ncbi.nlm.nih.gov/pubmed/20336685
Mary Ann Keatley, PHD, CCC, Laura L. Whittemore, Brain Injury Hope Foundation, Feed Your Body, Feed Your Brain: Nutritional Tips to Speed Recovery, Brainline.org,
http://www.brainline.org/content/2010/12/feed-your-body-feed-yourbrain-nutritional-tips-to-speed-recovery.html

S. L. Baker, New Study: Amino Acids Could Heal Brain Damage, Natural News,
http://www.naturalnews.com/027849_amino_acids_brain_damage.html

P. Simard, Ginko Biloba Promotes Better Blood Flow and a Healthy Brain, Natural News,
http://www.naturalnews.com/041535_ginkgo_biloba_brain_health_blood_flow.html

Lauren Saglimbene, Nutrition for a Brain Injury, Livestrong.com,
http://www.livestrong.com/article/35114-longtermeffects-trauma-brain/

Dr. Mercola, Fish Oil Cited in Dramatic Healing After Severe Brain Injury, Mercola.com,
http://articles.mercola.com/sites/articles/archive/2014/02/09/fish-oil-brain-health.aspx

Dr. Mercola, Tumeric Compound Boosts Regeneration of Brain Cells, and More, Mercola.com,
http://articles.mercola.com/sites/articles/archive/2014/10/13/turmeric-curcumin.aspx

Dr. Mercola, 9 Top Foods to Boost Your Brain Power,
http://articles.mercola.com/sites/articles/archive/2013/10/31/9-foodsbrain-health.aspx

Your Brain On Lentils: Depression-Fighting Powerhouses, All Treatment,
http://www.alltreatment.com/diet-and-depression

Mary Ann Keatley, PhD, CCC and Laura L. Whittemore, Brain Injury Hope

Foundation, Recovering from mild traumatic Brain Injury,
Brainlinemilitary. Brainline.org,
http://www.brainlinemilitary.org/content/2009/11/recovering-frommild-
traumatic-brain-injury_pageall.html

3-Therapies

Head Injury/Traumatic Brain Injury, YourSpine.com,
http://www.yourspine.com/Chiropractor/Pain+Issues/Head
+Injury.aspx

Gurley JM, Huisak BD, Kelly JL, Vestibular Rehabilitation Following Mild
Traumatic Brain Injury, PubMed.gov.
http://www.ncbi.nlm.nih.gov/pubmed/23648606

Vestibular Rehabilitation Therapy (VRT), Vestibular Disorders Association,
http://vestibular.org/understanding-
vestibulardisorder/treatment/treatment-detail-page

Vertebral Subluxation, Wikipedia,
https://en.wikipedia.org/wiki/Vertebral_subluxation

Andrea B. Ryan, The Role of Chiropractic in Traumatic Brain Injury: A Case
Study, https://www.torquerelease.com/pdf/011.pdf What is
Chiropractic?, WebMD,

http://www.webmd.com/pain-
management/guide/chiropracticpain-relief

Post-Concussion Syndrome: Why Isn't My Brain Working? Portland
Chiropractic Neurology,

https://www.portchiro.com/blog/article/2015/2/9/post-concussionsyndrome-why-isnt-my-brain-working/

Koren Specific Technique, Wikipedia,
https://en.wikipedia.org/wiki/Koren_Specific_Technique

Koren Specific Technique, Ted Koren Seminars,
http://www.korenspecifictechnique.com/

Mary Ann Keatley, PHD, CCC and Laura L. Whittemore, Brain Injury Hope Foundation, What is Biofeedback and Neurofeedback?, Brainline.org,
http://www.brainline.org/content/2010/12/what-isbiofeedback-and-neurofeedback.html

5-Sight-Light Intolerances

Prism Correction, Wikipedia,
https://en.wikipedia.org/wiki/Prism_correction

The Irlen Method, Irlen, Where the Science of Color Transforms Lives,
http://irlen.com/the-irlen-method/

Theraspecs Details,
https://www.theraspecs.com/whytheraspecs/

Simon Baker, Flicker Free Monitor Database, TFT Central,
http://www.tftcentral.co.uk/articles/flicker_free_database.htm

Liquid Crystal Display, Wikipedia,
https://en.wikipedia.org/wiki/Liquid-crystal_display

Fundamentals of Liquid Crystal Displays-How They Work and What They Do, Fujitsu,
http://www.fujitsu.com/downloads/MICRO/fma/pdf/LCD_B ackgrounder.pdf

LCD (Liquid Crystal Display), Whatis.com,
http://whatis.techtarget.com/definition/LCD-liquid-crystaldisplay

Paul Stone, How Is Your TV Making Your Concussion Symptoms Worse, NRI Neurologic Rehabilitation Institute at Brookhaven Hospital,
http://www.traumaticbraininjury.net/how-is-your-tvmaking-your-concussion-symptoms-worse/

Mary Ann Keatley, PhD, CCC and Laura L. Whittemore, Brain Injury Hope Foundation, Recovering from mild traumatic Brain Injury, Brainlinemilitary. Brainline.org,
http://www.brainlinemilitary.org/content/2009/11/recovering-frommild-traumatic-brain-injury_pageall.html

7-Exercise

Anish, Eric J. MD, Exercise and Its Effects on the Central Nervous System, Current Sports Medicine Reports,
http://journals.lww.com/acsmsmr/fulltext/2005/02000/Ex ercise_and_Its_Effects_on_the_Central_Nervous.5.aspx

Heidi Godman, Regular Exercise Changes Brain To Improve Memory, Thinking Skills, Harvard health Publications, Harvard Medical School,
http://www.health.harvard.edu/blog/regular-

exercisechanges-brain-improve-memory-thinking-skills201404097110

Benefits of Wobble Board Exercises, Sports Injury Clinic, http://www.sportsinjuryclinic.net/rehabilitationexercises/lower-leg-ankle-exercises/wobble-boardexercises

Brain Exercises for All Ages, Morsch Family Chiropractic, http://www.westfamilychiropractic.com/brain-exercisesfor-all-ages

53849875R00093

Made in the USA
Columbia, SC
21 March 2019